KEEP YOUR BREASTS!

Preventing Breast Cancer the Natural Way.

by
Susan Moss

First Edition 1994
Printed in the United States of America
Library of Congress Number 94-92245
ISBN 0-9642329-1-X

Publisher's Cataloging in Publication
(Prepared by Quality Books Inc.)

Moss, Susan.
    Keep your breasts! : preventing breast cancer the natural way / Susan Moss.
        p. cm.
    Includes bibliographical references and index.
    Preassigned LCCN: 94-92245
    ISBN 0-9642329-1-X

    1. Breast--Cancer--Alternative treatment. 2. Cancer--Alternative treatment. 3. Breast--Cancer--Prevention. 4. Cancer--Prevention. 5. Naturopathy--United States. I. Title.

RC280.B8M67 1994   616.99'449
                                          QBI 94-1640

Note to Reader: This book is for educational purposes only. It is not a substitute for a trained physician. The reader is advised to see a doctor for any physical problem.

The author and publisher cannot assume responsibility from the use and application of any information presented herein. There is no guarantee of cancer prevention or survival.

Front cover: "Night Sky" - oil on linen
7'x6' - 1991-2 Susan Moss

Back cover: "Green Peace" (for Kimberly) - oil on linen
6'x5' - 1993 Susan Moss

In Celebration of the Fifth Printing

"All women considering any form of breast cancer treatment should read this wonderful book."
—Deepak Chopra, Author "Path to Love"

"We plan to add your book to our permanent library which is utilized by our investigators and the university at large.
—Christine Wade, Research Manager
College of Physicians and Surgeons
Columbia University, New York, NY

"You write very well, and you are telling a critically important tale. Thanks for writing your story and thanks for living it."
—John Robbins, Author "Reclaiming your Health"

"We want you to know you share in our miracle."
—Brett Butler and his wife Eveline Butler
Cancer Survivor and L.A. Dodger Centerfielder

"It is outstanding that your book is already going into the fifth printing. I wish you all the best and continued success."
—Dr. David McFadden, Chief Surgeon, UCLA

"I want to thank you from the bottom of my heart (clichéd as that sounds) for your book. It must have taken a lot of courage and insight, not to mention time and patience, to pass this vital information to other women, gleaned from your own terrifying personal experience!

"I found the book serendipitously a few weeks into my own major breast cancer scare/emotional meltdown and it helped tremendously."

—Francis R. Ferrucci, writer, Los Angeles, CA

" *Keep Your Breasts!*' is a wonderful book about preventing breast cancer the natural way. Backed by extensive research, it talks about the fears Susan had to face, and how she went about taking control of her life and health, rather than letting herself become a victim of her lumps.

"Written with sensitivity and humor, the book also details the potential destruction that can accompany AMA endorsed treatments. Every woman should own a copy."

—Bera Dordoni N.D., Author "I Have a Choice?!"

"If you are strong, there is no precedent."

—F. Scott Fitzgerald

Table of Contents

Foreword

By Dr. James R. Privitera

Death from breast cancer as well as other major forms of cancer continues to increase despite refinements in diagnostic techniques and therapeutic modalities. The old standbys such as surgery, radiation, and chemotherapy are still used extensively. Many patients still receive the same toxic chemotherapy that was given thirty years ago.

Susan Moss beautifully chronicles the entire spectrum of diagnostic tests and treatments as well as the multifaceted causes and the most important personal point of view. She has an uncanny ability to separate the factual information from her own status as a "cancer" patient!

Certainly every woman who has a breast lump and anybody who has been told they may have cancer, should read this book since it differs from the others in being quite detailed in the causes of cancer, tests, pathophysiology, and loaded with recent information.

I have found this book to be among the best I have read.

I have practiced as a holistic health physician for over twenty years.

Acknowledgements

Thank you, Dr. Furr, for pushing the panic button that helped me to realize I had to save my own life! Thanks for suggesting I make the health program available to others.

Dr. David B. Clark introduced me to the Universe of the blood, spending many hours on its intricate workings.

Literary agent, Winnifred Golden, provided valuable guidance throughout, as did poet Michael Lenhart.

Editor Judith Regan, whom I met through the generosity of writer Paul Ciotti, provided almost as much encouragement to me as she did to Howard Stern!

Chuen Ng patiently taught me the computer. Special thanks for help to the UCLA Biomedical Library staff and Occidental College Library and Computer Center workers.

Editor Marion Philadelphia and screen-writer Arthur Sellers read and marked up the manuscript, making valuable suggestions.

Constant encouragement came from author Nancy Brinker, Nutritionist John Finnegan, Dr. Susan Love, Dr. Vicki Hufnagel, Meryl Streep, my niece Bridget Moss, my wise "health-nut" father, and supportive mother, Amy Moss.

To an unrelated "relative," Ralph Moss, for his information on cancer.

To Pam Kelly for coaching on speaking and giving me practice in her UCLA classes. Irene Lackey's many conversations helped me to edit my thoughts.

For Ed Siegler for friendship, encouragement, and legal advice.

Finally, to close the curtain, to actor Steve Martin for his incredible and uncanny ability to make me laugh myself well!

Introduction

You could see it all embedded in my genes, perhaps: the art, the psychology, the breast cancer. No one escapes the family. There was my grandmother, the painter, poet, and art collector who perished in the concentration camp before I could meet her. She became my spiritual guide. Remnants of her cousins, the Perls, art dealers and a psychologist, were buried in those microscopic bodily particles. On my Father's side, Aunt Rose, who had had breast cancer and a subsequent mastectomy she didn't talk about for years, contributed a more ominous DNA speck.

The programming was complete, deep within my bodily computer. Without knowing much about my relatives, I double-majored in art and psychology in college. My professor of psychology, Dr. James Nichols, and I established a suicide prevention center in the small university town where I lived. He wanted me to be a career psychologist. Driving past the campus grounds where I was sketching, he would shake his head. "Never forget your training in psychology," he admonished me.

I became an artist. Psychology was put on the back burner. Someday, I might find an urgent need to use it.

That day is here. I am putting down my brush—at least part-time—and picking up my pen to write about breast cancer.

My goal: to provide a breast cancer prevention handbook for all women.

Involved in creating with paint and crayons on large-scale surfaces of canvas and paper and showing the results around the country, I never had time to think about the disease. I never actually associated myself with it. Cancer was something that happened to "other people."

As I approached that age in which breast cancer usually strikes (forty-seven to fifty-three) it finally dawned on me that I was a high-risk individual. So I began doing research on the subject. I love personal stories. I read the autobiographical accounts of cancer by Jill Ireland and Gilda Radner. These women had everything: talent, beauty, successful careers, and adoring husbands. They could even write engaging, poignant books. When they became ill they could afford the best medical care: the best doctors, the most reputable hospitals, and the most cutting-edge treatments. Yet when I read these books, Gilda Radner was already dead of ovarian cancer and Jill Ireland was dying of breast cancer. Both women were still youthful, in their middle years. What was wrong with this picture?

Cancer was more of a mystery to me after reading these books than before. Modern medical science did not seem to be able to illuminate the subject and certainly the disfiguring and poisonous treatments they offered worked less than half the time. Some people only got worse, the trauma of the treatment actually shortening their lifespan. My aunt had survived her ordeal and was still alive, though minus a breast. For some people, surgery did seem to work. Why for some and not for others? And was there another path?

My father had been into holistic medicine for some time. He has always inspired and influenced me. Drugs and surgery had failed to cure his asthma and sinus problems. He found he got results from vitamins, health foods and practicing meditation to calm his nerves. He says he now regrets his decision to subject me to a tonsillectomy operation as a child of six years. He is now convinced that large doses of vitamin C would have solved the problems of my childhood illnesses. This is the only surgery I ever had. The indescribable suffering and anguish I experienced during and after that operation due to my raw, aching throat cured me of looking to a hospital visit to solve my health problems.

I was just as sickly a child after my tonsils had been removed.

I had a chance to try out my Dad's viewpoint later in life. After using acrylic paints for ten years, I became poisoned to the point that I developed a lump in the lymph nodes of my neck. I experienced shortness of breath, loss of appetite, and extreme fatigue. My weight fell off me several pounds at a time. I was an outpatient at UCLA for one year. Along with the medical treatment—a CAT scan which showed the lump, the Doctor telling me to give up using paint that emitted fumes and warning me that I would have to have surgery to remove the lump if it did not go away—I began to develop a simplified health program. My Dad bought me a juicer. I juiced carrots every night. I ran on the beach. I rubbed the lump with a fresh-cut lemon. Discovering visualization from a newspaper article about the work of O. Carl Simonton, I began creating my own version of this magic tool which I used every morning. Turning on some music with a strong beat, I would visualize little men in white coats going down my throat with a large rope which they would proceed to tie around the lump. I would then pull the rope upward out of my neck and through my mouth to the rhythm of the music. Within a year, I got rid of the lump, much to my doctor's astonishment. I made the discovery that when the body is healthy and detoxified and the mind is determined and positive, lumps in the body will disintegrate. A healthy body rejects tumors—even cancerous ones.

In doing this task, it was of the utmost importance that the body and mind work together.

Years later I witnessed the brutality of the medical treatment for cancer when my close friend Kimberly, age 34, found a lump in her breast. Despite early detection and immediate treatment—mastectomy, chemotherapy, and radiation—her cancer continued to spread. The treatment, worse than the disease, destroyed her health and beauty. She was not cured of cancer.

When that day came when my genes exploded into action and I faced my own crisis—two tumors, one in my breast and one in my uterus and subsequent chronic illness—I found that I had an opinion of cancer and its current methods of treatment. A rather strong opinion, at that. I had seen the medical treatment and read about the medical treatment. Whatever cancer was, the mystery had not been solved by the medical establishment. There must be another way. And if there was, I was determined to find it. After all, I had some positive experience at tackling a lump in my body.

To buck the system takes courage. To put your life on the line, choosing the role of human guinea pig is way past risk-taking, treading the line of the fool-hardy. But Dr. Simonton who inspired my own efforts has written that the belief-system of the patient and those surrounding her are of the utmost importance.

I believed that if I stared down a breast and uterine tumor using my own will power, while diligently following a health program of my own invention, my body would heal itself. Whatever disease-process I would go through, and I did go through a very traumatic one, I would allow my body the experience. I would fight using only natural means to support my immune system rather than begin the mutilating and poisoning of medical intervention that often destroyed the patient. I realized that I might be facing death. By rejecting medical intervention, I might sacrifice my life. Yet whatever battle was ahead, I felt strong enough to face it. By putting complete trust in my body while doing everything I could to support it, I believed that I would heal myself. Both my doctor, Dr. Wayne C. Furr, and cancer specialist Dr. James Privitera have verified that the symptomatology of the disease I went through was, in fact, cancer.

My health program had to be as comprehensive as possible. The theories that cancer had a psychological basis, a nutritional basis, and was connected to how healthy and "in shape" I was, had to be taken into account in my plan. Most of all cancer seemed to me to be a spiritual disease. Loss of hope equaled loss of life. My immune system could only be as strong as my belief system. My responsibility in constructing the disease had to be investigated in order to orchestrate its de-construction. **I didn't believe, actually, that it was all genetic programming.** I had to face the reality of my life and see how I had opened myself up to disease. I had to find the cause. In order to do this I had to take a soul-searching psychological journey.

Fritz Perls, my third cousin, helped invent Gestalt Therapy. He believed that neurosis and various diseases could be attributed to repressed feelings such as anger. He saw afflicted individuals as being *out-of-touch* with themselves. His patients were encouraged to live in the "here and now," to tune into and listen to their feelings. But until I faced two tumors in my body with my doctor screaming at me to see a surgeon, I didn't see how his writings pertained to me.

My doctor, after complete obstinancy in refusing medical treatment on my part, gave me two months leeway and then watched in amazement as I "spontaneously regressed" both tumors in the alloted time. (It took an additional seven months to get well). After his initial shock, he had the idea of sharing my program with others. "Make a video," he suggested. "I'll show it in my office."

But first a book needed to be written for women. (Men can also benefit as they also get breast cancer, though in males it is much more rare.) A book about courage in the face of chronic illness, by not only myself, but others as well. A book about self-responsibility. A book which suggested to the reader not to look for an outside *cure*, but to look within to *heal*. To depend, trust, and support the intricate healing mechanisms of the body. To provide an outline on how to go about supporting the healing systems that routinely heal the body. If we learn to use them, we can heal any disease, even cancer. For what is spontaneous remission, after all, but the effect of the body healing itself?

I now believe that breast cancer is a preventable disease. I believe that breast cancer can be dealt with quite effectively by using entirely natural means to encourage self-healing.

The statistics are frightening. Worldwide it is predicted by the University of Toronto, Canada, that one-and-a-half million women will battle breast cancer this year; one-third to one-half will die of the disease. When I began writing, one out of every ten women in the U.S. contracted breast cancer. Mid-way it had changed to one-out-of-nine! As I finish this project, only two years later, the rate is now reported as one-out-of-eight. Soon **all** women will be highly susceptible to encountering this potentailly lethal disease. Last year, forty-six thousand American women died of breast cancer. The disease now competes with lung cancer as the leading cause of death in women aged thirty-five to fifty.

Yet fear can now be replaced with a plan of self-care. I believe that if women would take my program to heart, modifying and personalizing it to fit their own lives, we could begin to reverse this negative trend. Women, armed with the information I gleaned from my struggle and from a year of research at the UCLA Biomedical Library to verify my conclusions, could drastically cut down their risk of becoming another fatality. This program may also help prevent recurrence for those that have already had an encounter with the disease.

My research included finding other women who had healed themselves, either with or without medical intervention. Their stories are a welcome addition.

Alternative, holistic medicine, once relegated to the corner of the health-food store is just now coming into its own. The National Institute of Health has just opened an office for alternative medicine. I believe holistic medicine is the medicine of the future. Amputation, poisoning with toxic drugs, and burning the body with radiation as a cure for disease will become archaic oddities of the dark ages of the past.

It's time to arm ourselves with knowledge. This book is about keeping our breasts and keeping our health.

No Time To Cry 1

Every woman's nightmare unfolded into the harsh light of reality one December day in the sterile cubicle of my gynecologist's examining room. Just a routine examination, or so I thought. But the atmosphere became charged with danger when the stone-like lump he found in my left breast near the nipple startled him into an emergency mode. He emitted a startled "uhh!" as if he had just touched a hot stove.

He had me put the first two fingers of my right hand on the lump. I felt the stone-like rounded mass, like a marble, on the inside portion of my breast near the nipple. Were my worst fears coming true? Did I have cancer? Would I have to have a mastectomy? Would I die?

My first reaction was denial. This couldn't be happening to me! I assured him I had lumpy breasts and this was nothing out of the ordinary. I have small, dense breasts. They have always felt lumpy in both self-examinations and physician-conducted ones.

He wasn't convinced. He told me that he had palpated many breast lumps and that this was no ordinary type of lump. It was something we had to investigate immediately. He also found a tumor in the upper left portion of my uterus adding to his anxious reaction.

I agreed to have a mammogram, overruling my serious reservations about this procedure which had, in the past, kept me from having one. Besides the damaging X-rays (even "low dose" X-rays have a cumulative detrimental effect) mammograms have an accuracy rate of only eighty-five percent. Fifteen percent of the time they are wrong. (According to Marie Zinninger of the American College of Radiology.)*

Kimberly had had a mammogram in 1989. It had come back negative, yet a subsequent biopsy showed she had cancer.

However, taking my doctor's advice, I had the nurse schedule one for me at the local hospital.

Because my left breast was diseased, and because my breasts are small, the mammogram proved to be both tortuous and injurious. My breasts were squeezed, squashed, and slammed between two metal plates by a technician. The pain was so great, I screamed bloody murder. The

---

*A blood test AMAS is available that is 95% effective at finding cancer. Call 1-800-9CA TEST.

technician had to re-do the procedure as the plates weren't clear enough—adding insult to injury. She hinted that, though it wasn't her role to tell me, there must be something wrong with my left breast as the procedure wasn't usually so painful. Both breasts were in severe pain for months after this routine X-ray screening.

My mammogram report came back negative.

Yet within one week I received a telephone call from my normally calm and controlled gynecologist. With utmost urgency, he said, "I want you to see a surgeon!"

Why was he discounting the painful procedure I had gone through? He seemed to be ignoring its findings.

"No!"

I repeated this negative stand throughout the next few minutes of our conversation.

After several tries to convince me, my doctor backed off. "Well come back into my office for a needle aspiration."

"No!"

I must have sounded like a broken record. To me cutting into the breast to determine its health was repulsive. Later, cancer specialist Dr. James Privitera explained to me the theory that a hard lump in the breast is the body's way of encapsulating cancer cells with a protein coating, and that cutting or poking into the breast opened the capsule, allowing malignant cells to spread into the bloodstream. I wasn't going to let this happen. If I had a lump, even if it was cancerous, I would figure out how to get rid of it myself. After all, I had done it before. I had practice returning my body back to health by physical detoxification and by utilizing mental imagery.

As an artist, the practice of visualization is very natural to me. When facing a blank canvas, or blank sheet of white paper, the first thing I do is start to visualize something that is not there. Then I proceed to "make" it appear. In order to do this I have to have faith and expectation, the confidence that I can accomplish this feat. Visualizing the disintegration of a lump in my body seemed to be about this process, only in reverse. I had experimented with this method in 1979. It had worked for me then. (In Chapter 8 I will explain how I used visualization to heal my body and keep it clean and free from tumors).

I was confident that I would be able to remove any lump from my body by myself, even a breast lump and the uterine tumor. If I had cancer I'd rather not have that diagnosis staring me in the face. I would just have to work harder.

Realizing my determination, my doctor relented.

"Well, at least come into the office within two months and have another breast exam."

"O.K." I told him. "I will do that. I'll call your nurse and set up an appointment."

I felt shaken when I put the phone down. What was I doing? Was I risking my life by bucking the medical establishment? To me, surgery is no cure for disease. In my opinion surgery has always seemed to be ninety percent fund raising activity—mainly benefiting the affluent lifestyle of the doctor. Cutting a pimple off your face is not going to cure you of acne. Another pimple will appear in the same place or nearby or somewhere else. Cutting the bumps off your body would not cure you of Chicken Pox. Lumps, bumps, and tumors which the body grows are symptoms of illness and/or the degeneration of the body. Cutting these symptoms off won't always work. The cause of the problem is not being attacked. My problem involved more than just a lump in my breast and a tumor in my uterus that could be surgically removed. Surgery would not magically change the conditions of my life. Whatever problems I had in my life—my diet, my environment, my emotional and business life—would still exist after surgery.

Still, the doubts crept in. I had "early detection," stressed by the medical experts as being so crucial. Was I gambling away my life?

I remembered the title of Betty Rollin's book on breast cancer *First You Cry.* I had every reason to break down into tears. As a matter of fact I could have bawled like a baby. I was terrified! But I couldn't afford the time to cry. I couldn't waste any energy on self-pity. Throughout my life as an artist I have been an independent, self-reliant person. I always met a challenge with all the determination and creative energy I possessed. I never had the luxury of time for feeling sorry for myself or for the victim role. Now I had my work on self-healing cut out for me and I had to roll up my sleeves and get to work.

I thought about my friend Kimberly. She had gone to "see the surgeon." She had early detection, seeing her doctor three days after she discovered the lump and immediately went into surgery. Her beautiful breast was removed. She was given massive doses of cytoxic chemotherapy until she lost her luxuriant head of strawberry-blond hair. She received radiation until her skin almost burned off. Two broken rib bones resulted from excessive radiation treatments. At age thirty-four, she began life as a "cancer patient with a malignant breast lump" and now at age thirty-seven, three-hundred thousand dollars in medical bills later, she still battles the disease which metastisized into her lungs.

That treatment simply was not for me. I had to find a natural alternative, one that was not mutilating and harmful. I had watched Kimberly being victimized and destroyed, her beauty and femininity taken away, not by her cancer but by the medical profession and their "treatments." I felt anger at the medical establishment. This fueled my own self-determination not to submit myself to any of these procedures. Why did they keep giving her chemotherapy and radiation when she obviously wasn't responding to them?

I visited the local library and book stores and loaded up with books on the subject of treating cancer holistically using natural means. Somewhere, there was the truth to be found that would enable me to get well using my body's own resources. I read books by Rose Kushner, Carole Spearin McCauley, Alice Hopper Epstein, O. Carl Simonton, Michio Kushi, Eydie Mae Hunsberger, Bernie Siegel, and Norman Cousins. These books which gave information on cancer and various holistic approaches, from eating raw foods to using laughter as an immune-system stimulant, formed my basic reference library.

When I began reading, the terrible truth hit me with full force. I **was** high-risk! "The Boston Women's Health Collective," for instance, described the age which most women encounter the disease—forty-seven to fifty-three. At the time my doctor found the lump I was forty-six and a half, almost right on schedule. Breast cancer seemed to coincide with menopause. My body was starting to go through a change although I had experienced no other symptoms. High-risk women also were Jewish and/or European, childless, single, and had breast cancer in their family: mothers, sisters, or aunts. Many also had had a lot of X-rays, used birth control pills, used DES, the morning-after pill, and had unhappy childhoods. Another psychological factor seemed to enter the picture: anger was a hard emotion for them to express and although outwardly they were cheerful and in control, inside they were churning with anxiety and emotions. High cholesterol also seemed to be a factor as was overweight.

All these factors applied to me!

I looked in the mirror and saw myself in a striped prisoner suit, labeled with, instead of a number, the words "HIGH RISK!"

I did have normal puberty, beginning menses at age fourteen (high risk is age twelve or under). Aunt Rose did not contract the disease until after she was eighty years old and had taken estrogen replacement therapy for twenty years (high-risk is first-degree relative with premenopausal breast cancer). Long term use of estrogens is being associated with a greatly increased risk of breast cancer. (See Chapter 2).

But other factors put me in the high-risk category. As an artist, I work with carcinogenic materials daily; the problem that had gotten me into health problems before. When I sprayed acrylic paint in the day, and breathed smog at night, I developed bronchitis which lasted six months. I have since eliminated fumes and air-borne particles but still use a variety of metal-derived pigments including ones with lead. Added to this fact is that I work each day in a smog-filled environment in the center of Los Angeles, California. This, too, has caused me problems in the past: severe allergies.

The picture, that of a middle-aged, slightly overweight, childless Jewish woman loner with financial problems and lumps and tumors in her body, was slowly forming in my book-clogged, anxiety-filled mind. No wonder I had problems! I was not only high-risk; I was headed for disaster if I did not find a way to change my life.

It had become clear to me why my health had been deteriorating in the past year. I had had a number of major set-backs that added up to big stress points if I were to plot them on a stress chart.

Financially my business producing and selling my paintings had taken a dive because of the recession. Despite having shows in New York, La Jolla, and Los Angeles, only one small work had sold. This oil on paper was purchased in La Jolla by a visitor from the East and my dealer had kept more than our agreed upon share to offset shipping costs. I had an emotionally tumultous on-and-off relationship with a highly intelligent, fascinating man. Emotionally unstable and unable to commit, he kept me at arms-length by constantly reminding me of his other girlfriends. This left me feeling abused and depressed. I recalled that when I had had the lump in my neck, I had also been going with an emotionally disturbed man who made me feel left out, jealous, and insecure.

My Los Angeles art dealer and I had also parted ways. A long-term successful relationship which included a close friendship, this blow had been particularly hard to take as it was entwined with my livelihood.

I had to take charge of my life and change it. Too many negative relationships, too much stress, too many problems were robbing me of my health. I would roll up my sleeves., create a health plan for myself, and follow it rigorously. Negative relationships had to go. Stress had to go. A detoxification diet and vigorous exercise program had to be begun at once. With a renewed sense of courage I took up my battle plan.

Still the doubts crept in. Was I taking too huge a risk? Would I simply die from "lack of medical intervention" in spite of early detection? Was I being strong-minded and stubborn or merely stupid? Did I have immense courage or was I making one huge tragic mistake? Would ignoring my doctor's advice to see a surgeon prove fatal? Would they simply write "we told her so" on my tombstone?

I decided after much of this agonizing debate with myself, to take a natural route, devising and following my own health plan as vigorously as I possibly could. I would give it two months to work.

What Causes Breast Lumps, Cysts and Tumors? The Triumph of the Weak Over the Weakened. 2

The breasts are the proud birthright of every woman. Aesthetically beautiful and mesmerizing in shape, they are the highlight of a woman's anatomy and have been celebrated since Adam first set his eyes upon Eve.

Figure one shows a sculpture by one of the first artists, a cavemen who lived in the region of Austria. This tiny fertility figure, only a little over four inches tall, emphasizes the huge, pendulous breasts of his model at the expense of the face, lower legs, and feet. We can see, by the process of elimination, what interested this caveman in his real or imagined model. Breasts have fascinated the human male for centuries and have helped us women attract and keep the interest of the man of our choice. A naturally nomadic man will return home, in part, for the pleasure of gazing upon his mate's breasts.

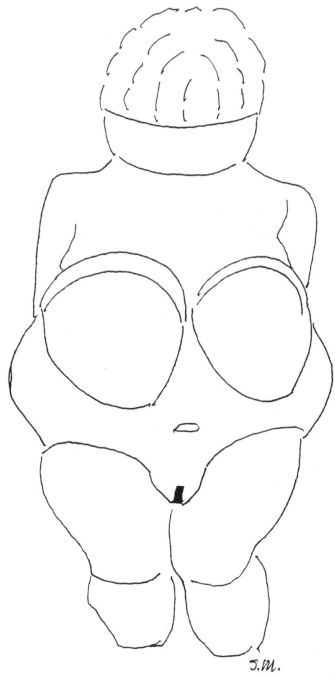

"Venus of Willendorf"

Figure One — Caveman Sculpture

Besides their natural function, to nurture and suckle the young with human milk (the best formula ever devised for infants), the breasts in their exquisite beauty have helped us in the economic world in getting jobs as actresses, dancers, and models. The power of their visual impact shows up in laws which prohibit us from exposing them in public and creates such a demand that men will line up to pay to see them.

We have only to compare the female human breast with that of other animals in the kingdom to see how fortunate we are. Think of milking a cow, or of how a cat or dog's teats look when these animals nurse their young. These bags of milk simply cannot compare to the stunning visual charms of the human counterpart.

Since we have such good fortune, it behooves us to become acquainted with its anatomy and functions as it prepares each month for the birth of possible children. We should learn how to do a thorough self-breast exam learning to distinguish normal lumpiness from a rock-like lump that may signal breast cancer is taking hold. Knowledge may enable us to learn to take care of our breasts so that they last the course of the lifetime warranty we should all have as a basic human right.

So let's look at the normal female breast. (Fig. 2). The breast is actually a modified sweat gland. It begins as a ridge in the fetus. At puberty it develops when the ovaries

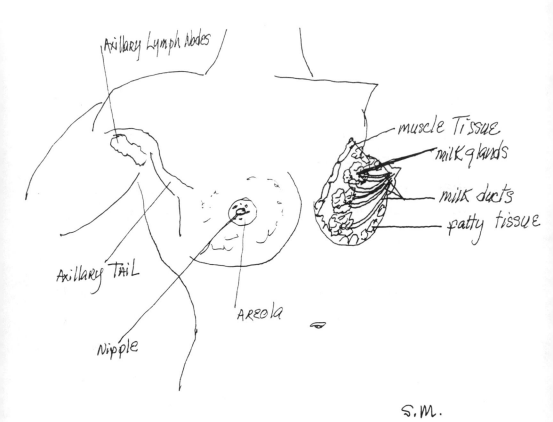

Figure Two: Normal Female Breast

send out a signal in the form of the female hormone estrogen. The branching of the duct system which carries milk to the nipple develops. Supportive tissues and fat construct the sculptural shape. Estrogen is responsible for making the areola a subtley darker color. The breast is not just frontal but curves around our ribs ending in a tail under the arm. The lymph nodes and tubes, carry white blood cells called lymphocytes that clean the breasts of impurities, viruses, infections, and cancer cells.

The lymph system is the body's garbage disposal system. The axillary lymph nodes (under the arm) are usually those involved first in breast cancer and where it is cleaned away from the body or may spread.[1] That is why, when doing the simplified three-step self breast exam I will describe in this chapter, it is also important to check for lumps and swelling under the arm.

The cells are arranged in clusters called alveoli. These enter into the milk ducts. The profound hormonal stimulus of pregnancy causes these cells to proliferate. The breasts then get much larger and nipples darken even more under the supervision, again, of estrogen. After suckling a baby, their main job, the breasts may grow smaller. With age they may either shrink and lose their suppleness, or they may become larger as breast tissue gives way to fatty tissue. Menopause continues the decline partly due to reduced

[1] Cowles, Jane *Informed Consent* New York: Coward, McCann, and Georghegan, Inc. 1976.

estrogen and progesterone production. ***However, each woman is different and may act in distinctly individual ways to their life-cycles.***

The breast is supported by two muscles located one on top of the other. These are called the pectoralis major and pectoralis minor which are also cleaned by the lymph nodes. In the Halsted radical mastectomy invented at the turn of the century for breast cancer, these muscles and some of the axillary lymph nodes were removed along with the breast. The excision of these muscles, which are used by the arm for a large range of motions, caused women major problems in restricting movement as well as leaving them with a concave, sunken-in look.

The breasts are ever-evolving organs. They are more than just milk factories. Their role in love and nurturing is of the utmost importance. Breasts are organs of emotion, of shape, of beauty. We need our breasts as they are an integral part of our femininity. How can we prevent problems? How can we keep our breasts youthful, elastic, and free from disease?

BREAST LUMPS

If we are to keep our breasts for a lifetime, we should check regularly for lumps. Normally, many breasts are lumpy especially right before, during, and after menstruation. Finding a lump is no cause to panic, as eight out of ten lumps are benign and non-threatening. A lump does not always signify cancer. However, we should note any lumps we normally have, so that if one appears that is "different" we can immediately consult our doctor.

Even if you find a lump, you can still get rid of it yourself. (This is what this book is about and how it differs from other books on this subject.) Surgery is not our only recourse.

The fact is the body is a self-healing entity. There are at least ten different types of white blood cells which we can empower to eliminate cancer cells.

Here, then, is an easy three-step breast exam. I have compiled it from several breast exams plus my own additions. Do it once a week—more if you feel there is a problem. You can incorporate it into your exercise routine, in the sauna, or in the shower at the gym or using a mirror at home.

STEP ONE: VISUAL. Stand in front of the mirror with breasts exposed. Examine your breasts and note any changes. Does one breast look different from the other? An inverted nipple may have been present from birth, but if it suddenly appears, this may be a sign of cancer. If one breast has a red or inflamed or swollen-out-of-the-ordinary look, this breast could be fighting a battle with cancer. Watch for nipple discharge. Some are normal. Others, like bleeding, could indicate trouble.

STEP TWO: PHYSICAL. With arm upraised use the first two fingers of your opposite hand to palpate or feel in a circular pattern around the breast. Start by going around the breast in ever-widening circles until you've worked the whole breast. Look for a lump that is different. Include an under-arm search, as lumps in this area may indicate trouble. You can also perform this exam lying down.

STEP THREE: MENTAL. Relax. Let your mind scan the inside of your breast. Do you sense any tightening or puckering? Is there any pain? Just go around your breasts using visualization to "see" what your breast normally looks like. Use your brain as an imaginary scanning device. Anything unusual? Is one breast hot or do you experience sharp, stabbing pains? Do you feel any pinching? How about stiffness or unusual hardening? Lift your arm a bit from the elbow and check for stiffness. You can imagine a white laser beam and aim this beam at your breast. Clean it with your light. Go around the breast as if you are cleaning your house in your imagination.

Your breast exam is done.

This version of breast examination is different from others because I have added this very important third step. This scanning technique may seem unusual, but think of how you listen for signs that something is wrong with your automobile. The slightest odd clicking and we head for our mechanic at the local garage. Yet paying attention to our body is something I often couldn't find the time to do. In the hurry and stress of modern life, our body may be trying to tell us that something is wrong. Our body may be breaking down, yet we haven't time to pay attention to it. We ignore it.

NATURE WILL TELL US WHEN SOMETHING IS WRONG. BUT WE HAVE TO TAKE TIME TO LISTEN.

There are many types of lumps we may find. Most of these lumps are benign. (Many women have lumpy breasts or their lumps come and go at different times of the month.) Some lumps that are non-threatening include fibro-adenomas which are composed of fibrous and glandular tissue and are rubbery, moveable, and painless. Cysts hold a watery fluid and are not cancerous. Ductal Papilloamas grow in the ducts close to the nipple. The mammary ducts can also become clogged with fat, creating lumps; or they can be clogged during breast-feeding.

A cancerous lump is usually hard, stone-like, and fixed. It would be located in the cells lining the milk ducts or in the lobes where the milk is manufactured.

I have proven to myself it is possible to get rid of a lump without recourse to surgery. If only we know how, surgery can be avoided.

It's important that we know our body. This way normal lumps, ''fibrocystic breast disease,'' will not be confused with cancerous tumors.

WHAT ARE THE CAUSES OF BREAST LUMPS?

The cause of breast lumps and cancerous tumors are not as yet perfectly understood. But we have definite clues. So let's make a list of possible or proven enemies of the breast.

1. Smoking.
2. Abuse of alcohol and drugs.
3. Excess fats in the diet.
4. Overweight (even the "usual five pounds").
5. Refined white flour, sugar, and their products.
6. Caffeine (chocolate, coffee, cola).
7. Birth-control pills.
8. Estrogen replacement therapy.
9. DES (the morning-after pill) banned as a drug to prevent miscarriages. Presently added to the feed of (or implanted in) chickens and cows to fatten them up.
10. Chemicals, additives, and plastics sprayed on fruits and vegetables. (Yes, plastics!)
11. Silicone-Gel Breast Implants.
12. Preservatives in foods, Nitrates.
13. Smog and environmental carcinogens.
14. Radiation.
15. Physical, chemical, or mechanical injury or irritation.
16. High animal protein diet.

17. Unusually severe stress.
18. Emotional loss.
19. Feelings of helplessness or hopelessness over a long period of time.
20. Unhappy childhood leading to problematic adulthood.
21. Some viruses.
22. Depression.

Although breast cancer is twice as high in families in which mothers, grandmothers, sister, or aunts had the disease, according to Dr. Susan Love in a lecture given at UCLA, in September 1992, seventy to eighty percent of breast cancer patients have no risk factors. Later in this chapter I will discuss my list of possible causitive factors in greater detail. But first, let's investigate how, in the worst-case scenario, breast cancer develops.

We always think of cancer as a vicious, powerful killer that overwhelms the healthy body with its brute force. However, the cancer cell is actually a weak, misinformed misshapen cell which has been damaged; and whose pro-gramming has been thrown off. A healthy body produces trillions of cells every 120 days to renew itself with a fresh supply. Some of these cells may be immature or bizarre in appearance. These cells are quickly caught by white blood cells such as macrophages which circulate throughout the body and are destroyed by them. The captain of this white cell patrol is our brain. We actually, whether consciously or subconsciously, dispatch this patrol with our attitudes and emotions.

Suppose we have eaten some poison in the form of a food additive and, as a result, a cell is damaged. The DNA in the nucleus of the cell is damaged. This DNA carries genetic information as to what this cell is supposed to do and how it is to behave in microscopic particles within it called genes. The oncogene (onco is tumor in Greek) may be damaged to the point that the programming changes from "grow" to multiply recklessly, uncontrollably, regardless of the space of other cells or organs and take over.

This formerly weak cell then becomes a little Hitler who started out as a weak person who flunked out of art school and sets out to gain power over the body by rapid growth and destruction. In a healthy body cancer cells are regularly produced and regularly destroyed before they can set up a colony or tumor-base. We don't "catch" cancer from another person. We manufacture it within ourselves—and we all have the ability within ourselves to destroy it. **Cancer cells are rejected by a healthy body in experiments to implant them.**

But let's say we are not at our peak of strength. Perhaps things have not been going so well in our lives. We may feel the futility of our efforts to make a happy life. Too many things have gone wrong. We feel hopeless or helpless about our situation. We are now on dangerous ground. Temporarily we may feel life just isn't worth living. Subconsciously we block the white blood cell patrol which protects us. Extreme negativity deactivates or slows down the immune systems' activity. This patrol can also be overwhelmed by carcinogenic chemicals, drugs, alcohol, or cigarette smoke. We need to nurture it with a nutritious diet and positive attitude. Our failure to do so puts us at risk.

Suppose, then, our patrol is not working at full force for one of these or other reasons. A bizarre cell in our milk-gland duct or lobes finds a weakened place to rest. This cell immediately seizes its opportunity. It's a rude and asocial cell "in business for itself." Normally cells, which are by nature restless and nomadic, are very polite. If they meet each other they sidestep. This courtesy is carried out by a fluted membrane sensor. The cancer cell, however, has a greedy, selfish, and destructive disposition. Its nuclei is bizarre looking, enlarged, or deformed. If missed by a despressed immune system, the cell begins to grow rapidly disregarding the space of other cells. By the time it can be palpated in the breast as a stone-like lump, it contains a billion cells. It has by then gone through thirty "doubling" times (doubling means one cell reproduces making two, then two make four, etc.). The cancer is on its path to destruction. After forty-three doubling times the patient may be dead.[2]

---

[2] Ibid.

This fact illustrates the ruthlessness and quick progression of the disease. However, the speed of growth is different in each individual. Slow growing tumors may be around for years, the immune system managing to hold them in check.

Still, this explains the emphasis on early detection and the anxiety of doctors when they find a lump. They have every reason to be alarmed.

The one cell that "got away" from our surveillance patrol, multiplies into a tumor and begins to set up its own blood supply. It then expands its "franchise" by the process of metastases, throwing out new versions of the crippled cell into its neighbor the lung or travelling through the bloodstream or lymph nodes to other remote parts of the body to set up new colonies, for instance in the liver or bones. In these new sites they like-wise invade and destroy.

A woman who has a cancerous, hard breast lump which she ignores, may go through the following: The cancer cells spill out of the breast lump and invade the skin fusing them together like a glue of destruction. The breast becomes rock-like swollen and red. (I actually went through this stage. Also my left arm became very stiff and difficult to lift indicating the involvement of the lymph nodes under my arm.)

If the cancer continues to grow it then destroys the skin. An ulcerated sore is all that there is left. It is rotten, infected, and smells putrid. The sore produces puss and sometimes

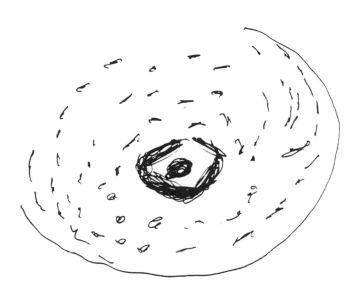

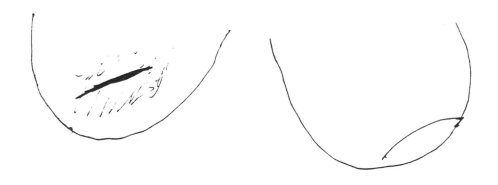

Figure Three: Signs of Breast Cancer

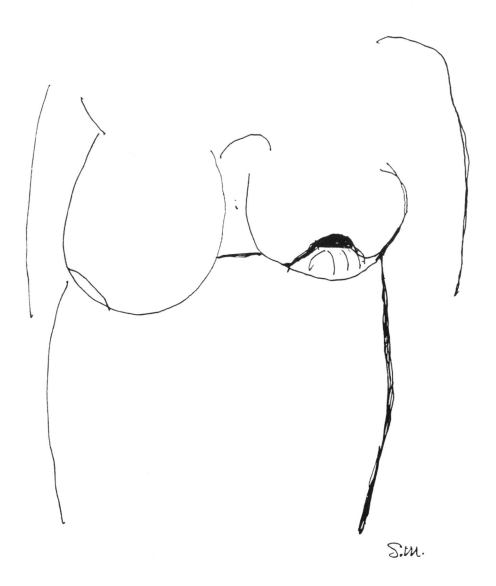

Figure Four: Advanced Breast Cancer

bleeds. By this stage the patient is truly suffering. Her breast is rotting. A coma may even be the result at this stage of disintegration.[3]

Fortunately, I was able to reverse the progress of my illness before this stage occurred although my breast did start to rot. It is an unbelievable stench, an odor I will never forget.

Once the cancer metastasizes to other parts of the body, the fight for life gets harder. The cancer begins to take over other vital organs, destroying them. The person may die of cachexia (wasting away of the body). Breast cancer is a gruesome disease. Thus it is in the best interest of all women to incorporate this list of "don'ts" into their daily lives.

1. **Smoking:** The World Health Organization's latest survey links deaths in the industrialized countries to cigarette smoking at 1.8 million per year. Smoking destroys the self-cleaning mechanisms of the lungs, paralyzing the small cilia that clean them. This paralysis is the major cause of lung cancer. Most lung cancers cannot be cured, although surgery, radiation, and chemotherapy can sometimes postpone death for six months to a year.

A study of 70-year-old women with first breast carcinomas [reported in the "American Journal of Epidemiology" (Jan.-Feb. 1990)] found cigarette smoking positively linked to fibrocystic breast disease (benign breast

---

[3] Ibid.

tumors). Another article in the same Journal ("Cigarette Smoking and the Risk of Breast Cancer") by Susan Y. Chu, Nancy E. Stroup, et. al.) reported a growing evidence that smoking has a definite effect on estrogen-related processes and diseases. Women who smoke had earlier natural menopause and an increased risk of osteoporosis (hollow bone disease), skeletal atrophy. A study of U.S. women aged twenty to fifty-four showed that those who reported smoking at some point in their lives had a higher risk of breast cancer than never-smokers. There was little difference between current and former smokers. The association of breast cancer with smoking tended to be stronger among younger women.[4]

In older women the anti-estrogenic effects of smoking in postmenopausal women were counter-balanced by other carcinogenic effects of smoking. Passive or secondary smoke has also come under scrutiny as possibly increasing risk.

Cigarettes contain tar, a known carcinogenic. Carbon monoxide produced in cigarette smoke robs the cells of much needed oxygen. **One theory of these bizarre cells is that they are regularly deprived of oxygen resulting in deformity.** Cigarettes are also preserved with formaldehyde, a known poison. The breasts are the lungs' neighbors. Often

---

[4] Weinstein, Bernard *Cancer Prevention: Recent Progress and Future Opportunities.* "Cancer Research" (Supp.) 51, 5080-5085 Sept. 15, 1991.

breast cancer will spread first to the lungs. It seems logical then that what damages the lungs will soon damage the breasts. Of course, if you die of lung cancer first, your breasts may still be intact at the funeral.

2. **Abuse of Alcohol and Drugs:** Alcohol is positively associated with a cancer of the skin called melanoma, a deadly cancer. For breast cancer, the association with alcohol was highest for women who drank one glass of beer daily and lowest for women who drank one glass of wine daily in a study reported in the "American Journal of Epidemiology." In a study of 90,000 nurses, excess risks often were apparent at relatively low levels of consumption—three to nine drinks a week.[5]

Drugs suppress the immune system, leading to disease and possibly cancer. We need a strong immune system at all times to ward off viruses as well as deformed cells. Why take chances?

3. **Excess fats in the diet:** "Time" magazine, Jan. 14, 1991 reports that high-fat diets promote the growth of mammary tumors in laboratory animals. Countries with low-fat diets have the lowest breast cancer statistics (Japan with one-eighth the breast cancer rate of the U.S.) Highest breast cancer rates show up in countries with high-fat diets: the U.S., Great Britain, and the Netherlands, while countries with low fat diets such as Japan, Singapore, and Romania have the

---

[5] Blot, William J. *Alcohol and Cancer* "Cancer Research" (Suppl). 2119-2123 Apr. 1, 1992.

lowest. When Japanese women adopt an American diet, their breast cancer rate soars. Japanese and American researchers are convinced of this high-fat, high-risk link.

4. **Overweight (even the "usual five pounds")**—A widower I met explained that he was depressed because his wife had recently died of uterine cancer. When I asked him if she was overweight he said, "Just the usual five pounds." He had me over to dinner one evening with a group of his friends and fixed an extremely high-fat meal (he did all the cooking while his wife was alive). High body fat content is linked to both breast and uterine cancer. **A woman does not have to be overweight to have high body fat content.** Increased body weight is associated with postmenopausal breast and endometrial cancers. (Bernard Weinstein).

A recent television special on breast cancer showed most of the patients with either breast cancer or benign breast cysts and fibroadenomas to be obese or seriously overweight. One terminally ill woman was shown frying large slices of bacon for breakfast.

Laboratory animals with tumors showed tumor regression when put on a starvation diet. The "American Journal of Epidemiology" reports that "Obesity remained a significant factor in breast cancer after controlling other factors."

5. **Refined white flour, sugar, and their products:** Empty calories in these foods which have been stripped of all

nutritional value can lead to nutritional deficiencies. Deficiencies in vitamins have been linked to various cancers especially vitamin A in breast cancer.[6] One prospective study of serum beta-carotene levels and thirty-nine women with breast cancer showed beta-carotene levels that were twenty-eight percent lower than those of controls.[7]

6. **Caffeine (chocolate, coffee, cola):** Caffeine has been found by researchers at Occidental College to damage the repair mechanisms of the DNA.

It also damages the immune system according to nutritionist John Finnegan. When I called the Breast Center in Van Nuys, California, the one substance they could point to as a cause of breast cysts was caffeine. Fibrocystic Breast Disease can sometimes be eliminated by cutting out caffeine, according to Nancy Brinker in her book, *The Race is Run One Step at a Time.*

7. **Birth Control Pills:** Hormonal pills alter the delicate hormonal balance of the system. Studies now suggest there is a fourfold increase of breast cancer in young women due to birth control pills. Two reports from Southern California (Pike, et. al. 1981-1983) suggest an increased risk of breast cancer in young women associated with oral contraceptive use either before first full-time pregnancy or before age

[6] Airola, Paava, Cancer—*Causes, Preventions and Treatment.* Sherwood, Oregon. 1972.

[7] Wald, N.; Thompson, S.G.; et. al., "Serum beta-carotene and subsequent risk of cancer." British Journal of Cancer. 1988 57: 428-33.

twenty-three.[8] Some of these pills feature estrogen and we know that estrogens enhance the growth of mammary tumors in mice. Others feature progesterone, and as Rose Kushner reports in *Alternatives,* a study of 314 Los Angeles women who used progesterone pills for birth control had a quadrupled risk of breast cancer after using these oral contraceptives for five years or more. Hormone-related cancers account for more than forty percent of all newly diagnosed female cancers in the United States according to Malcolm C. Pike, noted researcher in the field.

8. **Estrogen Replacement Therapy:** The "Los Angeles Times" April 17, 1991, reports, "The hormone estrogen that millions of women take to offset menopause symptoms may cause nearly five thousand new cases of breast cancer each year," government researchers report. According to the Center for Disease Control in Atlanta, the article went on to say, "Based on estimates of at least three million U.S. women taking estrogen, 4,708 new breast cancer cases and 1,468 deaths from the disease may be caused annually by estrogen use."

Usually prescribed is a pill called Premarin which is derived from pregnant mare's urine. Lying under a pregnant horse might be a more natural way to obtain Premarin! This pill is especially dangerous when taken over a long period of time, ten years or more. It is supposed to help prevent

[8] Pike, M.C.; Chilvers, C. "Oral Contraceptives and Breast Cancer: the Current Controversy" Journal of the Royal Society of Health. 1985 1: 5-10.

osteoporosis, but this can be done naturally with calcium in the diet and weight-bearing exercise. A popular notion is that estrogen will help prevent heart disease. This may be refuted by recent research into artherosclerosis in which calcium deposits, bone tissue, was found to be blocking the arteries of cadavers (patients who had died of this disease). Estrogens encourage the body to produce more calcium. Perhaps it goes into the arteries as well as the bones. If so, Estrogen replacement therapy could *cause* heart problems. (Dr. Linda Demer, "Journal of Clinical Investigation," April, 1993).

Taking estrogens will not keep us young. (At least Ponce de Leon was looking for FRESH water!)

My friend Cheri avoided the symptoms of menopause with Chinese herbs such as ginseng and dong quai and acupuncture. Other natural foods that contain estrogen are cucumber, sarsaparilla, soy products, and licorice bark. These certainly are worth a try.

9. **DES:** This synthetic hormone (Diethystilbestrol) was invented in 1938 and was known to be carcinogenic causing breast cancer in mice. Nevertheless, the drug was sent out into the marketplace where it caused considerable damage. Women who were given DES prescribed by their doctors as a preventative for miscarriage often developed breast cancer and their daughters developed vaginal cancer. Often they were born with deformed genital organs.

This synthetic hormone was further utilized to fatten up livestock and chickens and is **still** used today for this purpose. This is why American women cannot eat meat or chicken safely today. Twenty-one nations have a ban on the use of this chemical in food and 15 countries refuse to import American meat because of it (Paavo Airola, *Cancer the Total Approach*).

This hormone speeds up the sexual maturity in girls—one of the risk factors in breast cancer.

Tamoxifen, a drug given to cancer patients to prevent recurrence, and currently as an experimental drug to prevent cancer is a synthetic hormone derived from DES. Side-effects of this drug are possible endometrial cancer and liver cancer. Some studies show damage to the eyesight as well.

10. **Chemicals, additives, and plastics used on fruits, vegetables, and grains:** In this country the FDA allows twenty-eight hundred chemicals to be used on food and ten thousand more in their processing. Many of these are extremely carcinogenic.

When I was sick from the plastics I used in the studio, I discussed my condition with a number of chemists, to find out why my health had broken down. One showed me a hard acrylic sample about one-half by two inches. He proceeded to swallow it, telling me, "This product is perfectly safe. Why, they use it to spray apples and cucumbers!" He then went on to explain how they used to wax apples and other fruits and vegetables with beeswax but, it got too expensive.

To say that I was horrified when I left that chemist is to put it mildly. Go into any local supermarket and you will see very glossy apples and cucumbers as well as other fruits and vegetables. It is very important not to buy or eat these plastic-coated items. This plastic is hardened and will not scrape off or wash off. You might as well eat the plastic bags into which you put the fruit! Peeling is not good enough since skins are semi-permeable and the plastic gets inside. Eat and buy only mat or non-shiny vegetables and fruits, preferably organic. As we saw in the polyurethane-coated breast implants, the body attacks plastic and breaks it down to the chemical toluene, the turpentine-like solvent which causes liver cancer in mice.

11. **Silicone Gel Breast Implants:** Rivalling any macabre subject matter Edgar Allan Poe ever thought of writing about, the horror story of Silicone Gel Breast Implants is only now starting to come to light. Breast cancer and other degenerative diseases often have a long gestation period—twenty or thirty years or more. That is why only now (implants were introduced in the sixties) are the problems starting to surface.

Silicone Gel is an industrial material commonly used in the manufacture of electronic circuit-boards. With a catalyst added, it is marketed as a window and door sealant and ceramic tile caulking. Artists have used it as a paint medium. Recently I bought some to try but after reading the label, I decided the gel was too dangerous for studio use. (Contains ammonia and if gotten in the eyes call for immediate attention).

Silicone starts out as sand which is crushed and distilled in order to get silicone ore out and then reacted with methyl-chloride in a long process which eventually turns it into a heavy water-type liquid.

For breast implants this liquid is inserted into a bag of thin hardened silicone. This gel bag created immediate problems in women's breasts and bodies, such a capsular contraction, a hardening around the implant made of scar tissue as the body tries to wall it off. To solve some of these problems, a layer of polyurethane (plastic) coating was added to these bags of gel.

Often these bags would rupture or ''bleed through'' causing silicone gel particles to migrate throughout the body resulting in arthritic pain in the joints. Scleroderma, a chronic connective-tissue disease, and immune system disorders, where the body attacks itself (autoimmune) also resulted.

The polyurethane coating designed to stave off the hardened scar tissue (which plastic surgeons broke up manually in their office while the patient screamed and cried) is immediately attacked by the immune system which breaks it down in less than one year. The plastic is then further broken down inside the body to its component solvent, 2-toluene diamine (TDA) which has been linked to liver cancer in laboratory animals.

Toluene is a thinner much like turpentine only much stronger, that dissolves plastic. I would never think of using it in the studio!

Having worked with plastics for ten years and having been deathly sick for one year, I can testify first hand to the effects of plastics in the body; and I didn't implant them or eat them but merely got plastic into my system through breathing it and through the skin.

Plastic starts out as Rhoplex, a liquid plastic derived originally from petroleum, which was invented in 1910 by a German scientist, Otto Rohm, as a glue for cement. This plastic was kept in its liquid state, only made soluble in water by emulsifying the hard acrylic with ammonia. Once dry, however, it is no longer water soluble, which explains the body's quandary as how to get rid of it.

When I painted with the Rhoplex, it hardened up in one day or less, but as it did so it emitted ammonia fumes and formaldehyde, the chemical used as a preservative.

My symptoms were not unlike those of the women recently interviewed on KABC television who had had silicone gel breast implants, some of which had been plastic coated.

I became a "universal allergic" not being able to withstand any cigarette smoke even in a restaurant. Ink from a pen bothered me to the point I sometimes could not write a check. It took me one full year to recover after giving up plastics, and I only had a small amount of plastic in my body compared to the amount used to "texture" breast implants.

The women on the TV interview complained of chronic fatigue, joint pain, and lumps of silicone throughout their body. One woman had had five breast implants trying to find a new "improved" model that would not leak or create scar-tissue. A photo of her chest showed a roller-coaster of various deflated breast "shapes."

A photo of another woman's breasts showed a deep ulcerated sore one might see in a steadily advancing case of breast cancer. Interestingly she was the quiet one, seemingly apologetic and expressing no anger at her situation.

Still another woman who had subcutaneous breast surgery for cancer had had implants inserted which then ruptured. She then had new implants inserted. She complained of extreme fatigue and neuro-muscular auto-immune diseases.

Two million women have had breast reconstruction or breast augmentation using these unsafe industrial materials. These materials were never meant, in their inventors wildest dreams, to be put inside the human body!

12. **Preservatives in foods, Nitrates:** It's important to read labels. One breakfast cereal with a back to earth designed box contained preservatives. Children are especially vulnerable to these toxins. Fatty areas, such as in the breast, collect and store toxins. These are poisons added to kill mold. These poisons could also kill you.

Nitrates are found in processed meats and sausage. This chemical has been proved to be translated by the body into nitrosamines, which are extremely carcinogenic and can cause cancer anywhere in the body.[9]

13. **Smog and environmental carcinogens:** Exposure to air pollution in U.S. cities accounts for sixty thousand deaths annually according to a new study at Harvard School of Public Health. Many of these chemicals are carcinogenic. We badly need to clean up our air and water.

14. **Radiation:** New studies show that even low-dose X-rays can cause cancer over a long period of time. Even diagnostic X-rays used by doctors routinely have been implicated.[10]

Radiation is high-velocity atomic particles that destroy any part of the body at which they are aimed. Genetic mutations and cell aberation can result from exposure. Cumulative damage can occur throughout the body. One

---

[9] Aeola, Paavo.
[10] Dornfeld, J.M.; Thompson, S.K.; "Radiation induced changes in the breast": "Diagnostic Cytopathology," 1992, 8 (1) 79-80.

of the side-effects of radiation used in breast cancer treat-ment is further cancer years later, a case of today's cure being tomorrow's disease.

Another side-effect is seriously burned lungs leading to death.

Recently, a small vial of radioactive Cesium, a power-ful source of gamma radiation used to treat cancer and in food preserving, was lost somewhere in Northern Califor-nia. The "Los Angeles Times" (Feb. 24, 1993) warns that clutching the container would produce skin burns within twenty to twenty-five minutes, loss of hair within three or four days, and result in death after remaining in contact with the container for seven-to-ten days.

15. **Physical, chemical, or mechanical injury or irrita-tion:** Irritation of the skin over long periods of time can cause cancer. I saw for myself an example of how this can hap-pen. Sandy, the family sheep dog, used to chase cars, sometimes inadvertently hitting the side of his mouth against them. When he was eleven years old he developed cancer at that location of his jaw. Several operations failed to cure him; the growth returned after a short while. He could no longer eat and finally we had to have him put away.

In the course of my research, I met a nurse who in rushing to answer the phone, slammed her breast against the edge of a desk. She later developed breast cancer in that very spot. Although she also was going through extreme emotional turmoil at the time, she was sure that her injury contributed to her cancer. Her doctor, however, discounted it. This may be a cause-and-effect relationship overlooked by the medical establishment.

In another example, a pair of twins are highly studied by researchers because one developed breast cancer while the other did not. However, the sister with breast cancer had a physically abusive husband who beat her in the chest area.

Great care must be taken to protect the breasts from irritating fabrics or any sort of abuse or injury.

16. **High animal protein diet:** It is a myth that we need to eat a lot of meat. Meat and dairy fats are known to increase the risk of tumor development.[11]

17. **Unusually severe stress:** People with lowered ability to deal with the stresses of everyday life, those with worries and fears and severe emotional conflicts are more susceptible to cancer. The immune system shrinks when the body is under chronic, long-term stress leaving the system vulnerable to unchecked growth of mutated cells.

18. **Emotional loss:** High on the list of stress inducers are death of spouse, divorce, and separation. I witnessed this phenomenon myself. A neighbor of mine who at age sixty-two was a jocular, robust, healthy man, deeply devoted to his wife. When she died he radically changed. Dispirited

---

[11] Aerola, Paavo.

and confused, he seemed to waste away before my eyes and within two months this very healthy man was dead of heart failure.

In the same way women have also developed breast cancer after losing their husbands.

19. **Feelings of helplessness or hopelessness:** Loss of hope for a rewarding life and lack of enthusiasm for living creates depression. During a depressed state the immune system shrinks in size and begins to shut down.

20. **Unhappy childhood leading to problematic adulthood:** According to O. Carl Simonton, cancer often strikes those who feel rejected by one or both parents in childhood. When we are "thrown back" to that original feeling of rejection because of a current setback, we often cannot get back on our feet and the result is we can't protect ourselves from the bizarre cells that cause tumor growth.[12]

21. **Some viruses:** Although we can't "catch" cancer, one form of virus, the Rous Sarcoma was shown to cause cancer in chickens as early as 1910. There may be other viruses involved according to Dr. David B. Clark.

22. **Depression:** Loss of a reason to get up in the morning. Being at a loss as to know how to create a meaningful life for oneself becomes the psychological undermining of the body paving the way for cancer according to psychologist Dr. Lawrence LeShan.

---

[12] Simonton, Carl O., M.D. and Stephanie-Matthews-Simonton; Creighton, James L.; *Getting Well Again.* Toronto, Bantam Books: 1978.

As I write this book, women ask me why, if cancer has always been around, is there suddenly this enormous increase of incidence? My answer is pointing the finger of suspicion at high-fat animal protein diet, miracle hormone drugs, and plastic surgery on the breast which we believed would make life easier and sexier when introducd in the sixties but in creating disease have a twenty- to thirty-year latency period. We are just now seeing the tragic results of hormone pills designed to give us reproductive freedom and take away the symptoms of menopause: synthetic hormones given to livestock to make meat more commercially appealing: fruits and vegetables grown and sprayed with chemicals, poisons, and plastics; and the extreme stress contemporary women experience in trying to "have it all" (be mothers, full-time career women, and housekeepers all at the same time).

Let's look at the positive side before we close this chapter—what factors can help us to keep our breasts healthy:

1. A low-fat vegetarian diet.
2. Weight control—reaching and maintaining our ideal weight.
3. Positive attitude. Being happy. Enjoying our work.
4. Having children before age thirty and breast-feeding them.
5. Having a religious or spiritual practice.

6. Once a month fasting or under-eating for a day.
7. Learning how to handle stress so as not to take it out on the body.
8. Group therapy when we have problems.
9. Good marriage.
10. Expressing our feelings (especially not holding onto anger and resentment).
11. Limiting our exposure to X-rays, chemicals, and smog.
12. Regular vigorous exercise, preferably one hour a day, five or six days a week.
13. Regular self-breast exam, once-a-year breast exam by a gynecologist, and mammogram when a suspicious lump is found.
14. Turning down technological "miracles" that haven't had a twenty year follow-up study (such as birth control pills, estrogen replacement therapy, implants, and routine yearly mammograms).
15. Protecting ourselves from mechanical or physical injury.
16. Learning how to self-heal our bodies, including how to rid one's body of tumors by natural means.

In summary, KNOWLEDGE IS POWER. Instead of feeling anxiety about breast cancer as something that may strike us out-of-the-blue, we can be confident that there are definite causes and therefore preventative measures which we can incorporate into our daily lives. There are many things women can do to stay healthy and not become a cancer statistic. We can improve our chances of avoiding breast cancer. Pasteur once said, ``Chance favors a prepared mind.'' We can work on cancer prevention every day of our lives.

BE LIVING PROOF!

Who's The Boss? Making Your Doctor A Partner Rather Than An Authority Figure. 3

Dr. Furr (a good name for a gynecologist, I kid him), is a highly respected enormously competent doctor for whom I have the greatest regard. However, Dr. Furr knows that with me as a patient, he always gets a second opinion. And that second opinion is **MY** opinion.

Since most of his other patients seem to regard him with an almost religious awe and take whatever advice, pills, devices, and treatments he prescribes with little or no resistance, he tends to regard me as somewhat of a peculiarity. But, over the years, I have earned his respect.

When I argue with him or turn his suggestions down flat, he looks at me as if I am "something else"—for instance a visitor from some distant planet. Sometimes he has even laughed. Turning my doctor into a partner rather than a medical authority has not been an easy task, but a worthwhile one.

Yes, he is my doctor. Yes, he has a great deal of knowledge, wisdom, education, experience, competence, and success. But since this is my body he is treating, I have the final say.

Women who see themselves as the traditional ''second sex'' often have trouble dealing, in their everyday lives, with authority figures. Males still hold the power in our society despite inroads made by women. Eleven percent of our doctors and gynecologists are now women, and I have been to some. However, they were still taught by men. Although men can study, learn, and treat a woman's body, they can never really understand it because they are men. Women in our society are subtley conditioned to be sub-servient and to believe that we may not ever be as smart, powerful, or successful as men. We are often ready to accept a passive role when we visit the impressive offices of our doctors. Many times women decide merely to ''trust'' their doctors giving them carte blanche to prescribe whatever they think of, submit themselves to any diagnostic procedure, swallow any drugs, agree to have any part or organ surgically removed, and pay any exorbitant amount in the belief these things will benefit their health.

When we go into a doctor's office prepared to ques-tion, prepared to challenge, willing to do our own research into our particular problems, willing to take responsibility for our own health, willing to stand up to the male authority and/or the authority and power of the medical establishment, we find that we create the partnership it was meant, originally, to be.

My own experience of how I accomplished such a relationship with my doctor may be useful.

After my highly trusted and reliable gynecologist, Dr. Caldwell retired, I had a terrible time finding a replacement. Who can ever find a substitute for a long-standing relationship in which you felt the doctor really cared about your health? Also, Dr. Caldwell treated me for other problems and acted as my General Practitioner.

After making the rounds of HMO's, clinics, and other doctors and finding nothing but frustration, I found Dr. Furr, through a friend's recommendation.

He immediately impressed me with his skill and intelligence. On my first visit, he executed a Pap Smear using that horrid metal speculum, without, somehow, causing me any pain. This was a completely new experience and I was sold on Dr. Furr, happy that I had, at last, a new doctor.

However, I found over the years that I had to work hard on changing our relationship. Dr. Caldwell had been older and somehow was more open to opinions and discussions, always asking what I thought. Dr. Furr, perhaps because he was younger, was more into prescribing what he thought best, going by the rule book, and having the patient simply accept it. I felt that Dr. Furr was quite used to having control over his female patients. Therefore, a bit of quiet power struggle went on at times during some of my visits.

When he quoted the rule book, for instance, that because I was forty-five, I should subject myself to a mammogram every year, I balked. I told him I had gotten too many X-rays during my lifetime for various illnesses and injuries and that as long as nothing was wrong, I would rather postpone this procedure.

A new and yet unpublished study by the National Cancer Institute of Canada substantiates my instinctive belief that regular mammograms may be extremely harmful. This study followed fifty-thousand women ages forty to forty-nine between 1980-88. Half the women got diagnostic breast X-rays every year-and-a-half. The others received only physical examinations. Astonishingly the death rate from breast cancer in the mammogram group was significantly higher, by fifty-two percent!

I could tell he was not happy with this decision or the fact that I was asserting myself in the decision-making process; but a man of few words, he merely grunted and let me go.

The next tug-of-war came when, on another visit, he thought a newer model birth control device would be better and more effective than my old one. I took his prescription but I had rather severe problems with it. He wrote me another prescription for my old device which he sent into the pharmacy without further arguments. The biggest challenge came, however, when on my annual check-up in December 1990, he found a hard stone-like lump in my left breast. He became extremely nervous and anxious and I could tell this lump meant Big Trouble. Having often opposed Dr. Furr's advice, I saw now that it was time to take it.

Still, I knew that the big challenge to change our relationship was now upon me, I was going to have to make it clear to him that although I still needed him to be my doctor, I was in no way going to follow through, even if I had cancer, on the "orthodox" methods of treatment. *Still I want to emphasize that without Dr. Furr's finding my tumors, I might have died oblivious to the fact that I was becoming chronically ill.* Cancer is called a "silent killer" as often no symptoms show up until the disease is two-thirds of the way into its destruction. Often no pain or illness is felt for years. I felt nothing.

When he found the lump, Dr. Furr did not ask me any questions about my life. Was I under stress, for example? Was I worried or depressed? How was my diet? What about my emotional life? How was I sleeping? These questions were not asked.

After the mammogram, his next command and telephone campaign was, "I want you to see the surgeon!"

After I said "No!" enough times he finally understood.

I agreed to come into his office again in two months for another breast exam. Then I sat down and wrote him a letter.

It takes enormous courage and strength to stand up to the medical establishment, or even question their authority. But this is a job we women have to undertake. It's easy to feel intimidated and powerless in the doctor's office. It's easy to take the passive role and just do whatever he says.

However, we pay a high price for this unquestioning attitude. Following an authority figure with complete trust leaves us wide open for abuse.

Although my transition from traditional medicine to alternative has been gradual, I now object strongly to the mechanical nature of western medicine where the patient is basically treated as a robot-like creature whose illnesses and problems can be diagnosed with space-age machines like X-rays, CAT-scans, and MRI's which make you feel you are taking a trip to Mars; then the part of your body that is not working properly is either "corrected" with pills or removed with surgery. I object to the assembly-line methods of treating a patient where a part can be removed, replaced or fixed like a car. I object to the out-of-hand costs of such treatments that seem to spiral up every minute and to the concept of physicians being able to make increasingly larger sums of money while not always curing a patient or increasing his or her lifespan.

Iatrogenic, or doctor-caused diseases, usually the

domain of the malpractice attorney, are examined by Siegfried J. Kra, M.D. in his book, *Examine Your Doctor—A Patient's Guide to Avoiding Medical Mishaps.* His impetus for writing such a book came about when his Father was misdiagnosed when he collapsed on the street and died six hours later in the care of surgeons who treated him for the wrong ailment.

He points out that, next to lawsuits involving hospitals, the procedure most often paid in malpractice suits involves the treatment with drugs (between 1975-78). I think it's especially important, when a doctor prescribes a drug, to not only find out all about it, but investigate precisely what all its side-effects might be. I would even go a step further and find out if it is really needed or if there are natural foods or herbs that would work as well or better.

As a case in point, after spending hours researching at the UCLA Biomedical Library, I have piled up enough evidence against estrogen to condemn it as contributing to breast cancer:

1. Women who have their ovaries, which produce estrogen, removed before age thirty-five, are virtually free of breast cancer.
2. Estrogen resembles, in composition, a carcinogenic substance.
3. Obese women have been found to have higher estrogen levels and have more breast cancer.

4. Young women who have taken estrogen birth con-
    trol pills have a quadrupled rate of breast cancer
    according to British studies.
5. Estrogen replacement therapy may cause up to five
    thousand new deaths a year, increasing a woman's
    risk by at least thirty percent.
6. Some breast tumors actually set up estrogen recep-
    tors and are estrogen-dependent for their growth. Yet
    doctors continue to prescribe estrogen-based pills
    rationalizing that they are "low-dose." Among un-
    married women, the pill is now the most popular
    method of birth control. At least ten million women
    who are postmenopausal take estrogen replace-
    ment therapy pills unaware that they are increasing
    their chances of getting breast cancer.

Clearly, if the doctor we see has not gotten the above
messages, it is up to us to inform ourselves and communicate
with him or her.

Women I interviewed who are now suffering from auto-
immune diseases and other serious side effects caused by
breast implants talked about "trusting" the plastic surgeon
whom they went to for this procedure. That these implants
were never tested or approved in any way and that the
doctors' knowledge of the industrial materials supplied by
a chemical company was very limited or non-existent, was
never a subject explored by these suffering women.

Dr. Kra further lists malpractice suits from in-hospital events: "accidents involving anesthesia, transfusion mishaps (I think here of the recent AIDS contaminated donor whose organ donations affected the lives of fifty patients, killing many), procedural errors, as well as operations on the wrong patient or the removal of the *wrong organ*!" (My italics).

While I definitely want to keep Dr. Furr as my doctor, I feel the necessity to stand up to him and to do my own research. As an avowed "self-healer" who has experience getting rid of lumps and bringing myself back from various close calls, I favor an holistic approach. While not ruling out all pills (antibiotics are a great invention that occasionally I have resorted to), I favor vitamins over drugs, utilize vegetable and fruit juices, herbs, spiritual healing, group therapy, visualization, water therapy, rest, sun, air, and exercise in order to heal myself from within rather than rely on pills, surgery, or other drugs. As for birth control, barrier methods suit me best and these also act as barricades when used with spermicides against many sexually transmitted diseases.

Doctors take the Hippocratic Oath when they enter the profession; one of their pledges being they will do no harm. They also promise not to give fatal drugs to anyone.

Turning Dr. Furr into my partner in self-healing was another challenge. I accomplished this by "forgetting" when my appointment was to re-check my breast in two months. Having to call regularly amused the receptionist but gave me a repetition of the deadline my body had to meet. In this way, Dr. Furr became a motivator in my self-healing program. This is the only healing connection I had outside myself. It was very important to me. More important, in fact, than any drugs or surgery. He had found the lumps and had set up a deadline. Not that he believed that I would get rid of the lumps myself—that was what *I* believed. If anything, he probably had *disbelief.* This was not one of those benign types of lumps that merely disappear of their own accord. To rid myself of it took a total declaration of war; I fought one of the great battles of my life. I looked jaundiced. My energy seemed to have been vacuumed out. My body felt like it was disintegrating. My hair became stringy and lifeless, a wet mop. Fatigue, listlessness, and pain became my every-day experience. Finally, to my horror, my breast began to rot. Weird symptoms began occurring making my body grotesque-looking and immobile. Friends who caught a glimpse of me commented, "You looked really sick." "You looked *green.*" "You looked like death only slightly warmed over!" And at one point, I actually saw myself losing my life as my health began to slide downhill. Yet, I battled on!

The proof of the pudding of our medical system which relies so heavily on drugs and surgery, is life expectancy. Japan's life expectancy for women is the highest—82.5 years. That compares to 78.6 years for U.S. women.

Until 1968, Japan was a closed society and relied on

Chinese practices of medicines. The Chinese use herbs, macrobiotic diets, acupuncture, and other natural methods to help the sick. We lag behind the Orientals who have now adopted European and American "scientific" methods of cure to their detriment.

As I go through my life, I find myself relying more and more on ancient wisdom while turning away from modern technology with its "better living through chemistry."

In my work I turned away from plastic paints with their promise of quick results because they made me very ill, to the most traditional and historical of mediums—oil paints. I adopted an ancient ritual of Buddhism for my spiritual needs. It is a practice which originated in India, one of our oldest civilizations as filtered through Japan. When I am ill, I find myself rejecting modern technological advances which rely on external methods. In their place, I substitute ancient self-healing methods, relying on building inner strength by a slow biological process of internal healing. Any doctor will admit under cross-examination, that with all his treatments, ultimately the body must heal itself.

In our secular, existential, scientific age it's easy to forget that the doctor-patient relationship was originally tied to the Spiritual. Prehistoric people did not have doctors. They consulted priests. These priests offered prayers for the sick person. Disease, first and foremost, was considered to be spiritual in nature. Any "medicine" consisted of herbs which were found to have power to help the body heal. But primarily, the body healed itself—being invested with its own recuperative powers. With the help of the Spirit, the body did its routine job of healing. The ill person, then, was inspired to help himself.

Although modern medicine has helped raise our life expectancy by eradication of many diseases, and our better systems of hygiene have led to greater steps in prevention; we have seen no progress in the treatment of breast cancer since nineteen hundred thirty and the death rate has remained the same.

Hippocrates, the Father of Modern Medicine, was a priest who worked out of a temple, Asklepian Temple at Cos. Temples were located near hot springs with mineral waters which were used in the healing process. Treatment of the sick also consisted of rest, temporary abstinence from food, exercise, massage, and "temple sleep" in which dreams were interpreted by the priest, the origins of our psycho-analysis. If the patient did not dream, the priest created a dream for them to interpret. Mind and body were considered one; and the mind, which contributed to the illness, could also contribute to the healing. Psychological factors, before the term was invented, were considered to play an important role in disease.

Hippocrates saw cancer patients. It is thought that he invented the term carcinoma. Not being able to find a cure for the disease, he found that patients lived longest when left alone or given mild treatments such as applying poultices, and he forbade surgery for lumps as it harmed the patient. Above all **"Do Not Harm"** was his dictum.

Priestesses who helped heal in the temple were also available to the ill person. The legacy handed down from the Ancients—that the body heals itself from its own recuperative powers with only the help of what is now termed "alternative" methods such as herbs, nutrition, massage, rest, fasting, mineral water, exercise, dream interpretation, and prayer has had quite a struggle to survive when pitted against the giant economic monopoly of modern medicine with its emphasis on drugs and surgery and its male-oriented approach toward science, mechanical treatments and impersonal "objective" treatment of the patient.

Nevertheless, alternative approaches have survived mainly because they often work. Their practitioners, however, have had a terrible struggle, often for their life.

In early England most of the healing was aided by women healers who combined wisdom, nurturance, and herbs with counseling and who gave of their assistance and knowledge freely or with little money at stake.

On the other hand, a surgeon who unsuccessfully operated on a patient, for instance operating on an eye and causing blindness, was subject to having his hand cut off. Also, surgeons could be sued for overcharging.

Women healers did most of the work of helping to heal the sick, and were valued for their knowledge and skills. However, in the fifteenth and sixteenth century in Europe they were branded as "witches" and thousands upon thousands were executed, usually by burning at the stake. This happened during the Inquisition when the Medieval Church controlled medical education with its hierarchy of King and Princes and Authorities. The witch trials established the male physician as being superior morally and intellectually to women healers who were thus associated with magic and evil. This suppression of women and "alternative" methods of healing continued in 19th century America sans executions but instead with economic suppression.

Medicine became a commodity, a way for a male physician to acquire great wealth while female knowledge was passed down freely and practiced without charge as a neighborly service. Soon legal suppression of women healers and alternative methods arose.

In the 19th century, it was thought that laws should be passed prohibiting mid-wives to practice their art and they were accused of being "filthy and ignorant and not far removed from the jungles of Africa" (Underwood, 1926). This way birth became to be viewed as only to be administered and supervised by the male medical establishment.

Thus our present doctor-patient relationship has a long history of social and economic struggle. This struggle is reflected in our current philosophies in how breast cancer is currently treated which I will go into further in the next chapter.

But to conclude this one, I think it is of the utmost importance that when going to a doctor for a problem, to go with a questioning attitude, to form our own opinions as to what we will "buy" or "buy into" from our doctors.

It's our bodies, we know them best. Can our problems be solved with pills or surgery? Has the doctor made the correct diagnosis? Does he want you to take a test so as to avoid a malpractice suit? Can we stay out of the hospital? Would an alternative approach of self-healing give us better, longer-lasting results?

It's time for women to empower ourselves. In the end, it's our bodies. We're hiring the doctor to give us advice. We are the boss.

The Termite Theory
of Breast Cancer Treatment **4**

The treatment of any disease is based on a paradigm, or concept of the disease. Until the paradigm changes, the treatment cannot change.

The paradox of cancer is that there are concurrently two paradigms utterly opposed to each other and at war with one another: an orthodox medical establishment view vs. an holistic, alternative construct. However, officially and by law, the "orthodox" concept has won out without evidence, in the form of progress in cure or lowering the death rate, that it is approaching physiological truth.

Faced with the evidence that I might have cancer, a formulation of a concept of the disease was urgently needed in order to decide on a route of healing or treatment.

The orthodox medical establishment was insistently fixed

upon a notion that seemed at once absurd and antiquated to me: that cancer was a bug, like a termite, that could be treated by cutting, burning, and fumigating with poison chemicals. Statistically, this male war-like view of attacking cancer was not changing the death rate in breast cancer which actually went up three percent in the thirty years between 1955-1985.[13] Nor was it seemingly bringing insight into the disease as twenty years and billions of dollars spent on the war on cancer only produced the following announcements:

1. We don't know what causes cancer.
2. We don't know how to prevent cancer.
3. We don't know how to cure cancer.
4. But we do know how to charge for cancer.

Cancer treatment using the Termite-paradigm: surgery, radiation, chemotherapy, and bone-marrow transplants can now cost three-hundred-thousand dollars or more. Statistics in the success of such treatments showed no rationale for these tortuous and mutilating procedures or for the charges. Often worse than the disease itself, they were what actually killed the patient!

Statistics are one thing, but closer to home was my friend, Kimberly. Clearly there was something drastically and profoundly inaccurate about using "aggressive treatments" to enable surgeons to "get it all" thus removing the enemy

---

[13] Moss, Ralph, The Cancer Industry. New York. Paragon House: 1980, 1991 p. 26.
   Also see Chapter Two: "The Proven Methods."

bug and returning the body back to "normal" sans "termites" or cancerous cells.

I watched in horror as my friend, who caught her lump so early it did not show up on her mammogram, progressively lose her breast, her hair, her immune system. I listened to her describe inhumane, debilitating, neutering treatments which caused her unending hours, days, and weeks of vomiting and nausea, arthritis in all her joints from her implant, severely burned skin, and two broken ribs from excessive radiation treatments. I watched as she was transformed from a stunning, vibrant, and extremely beautiful and feminine young woman of thirty-four to a stark version of a unisex concentration camp victim three years later, grasping at life in a humiliating display of complete and utter devastation.

No! It was so easy for me to say "no" to this paradigm and subsequent treatments. It not only seemed wrong to me, it was grotesquely cruel. Convenient for the medical establishment, perhaps, as chopping off the breast, though it involved severance of many nerves and much bleeding, was relatively easy since the breasts are so conveniently out-front and this operation brought large financial rewards. Added to the enormous bill were the highly dangerous implants, toxic chemotherapy drugs, and radiation with its attendant risks of heart disease, broken bones, damaged skin, and risk of causing more cancer down the road. These abhorent methods, harmful and chauvinist to the extreme, worked in less than half of the breast cancer patients they attempted to cure. Other women might not question this violent approach, but to me, the idea that disease can be cut out of the body was absurd! Surgery, for me, was completely out of the question.

Historically, the radical mastectomy was invented by Dr. William Stewart Halstead a century ago. A "last-ditch" treatment for very advanced disease, it became the vogue though it only prolonged the life of twenty-five percent of the women who underwent this drastic treatment.

A painting by the eminent artist Thomas Eakins from that time, "The Agnew Clinic" illustrates well some of the quasi-scientific reasons for its popularity.

A gorgeous, shapely woman lies bare-breasted in a swoon on the operating table, her arms raised seductively over her head, helplessly succumbing. She looks ravishing and ready to be ravished. A suited, bespectled instructor watches calmly and authoritatively as a student surgeon proceeds to cut off one of her voluptous breasts. Surrounding this drama in the rounded theater, an audience of male students watches, leaning eagerly forward, their gazes transfixed and their eyeballs bulging out of their sockets.

A note of lewdness creeps into this work of art, unusual in the work of this artist known for anatomical mastery, precise rendering of detail, and classical subjects such as young men jumping into the local swimming hole. Perhaps part of the popularity of this operation is that it satisfied man's ambivalent feelings toward women. As for the patient, she died seventy-five percent of the time regardless of this "treatment."

In her *Breast Book*, Dr. Susan Love, a breast surgeon, explains, "If you look at the history of how we've dealt with any disease, you'll see that, when we don't yet understand it we do things like surgery."[14]

BEING SICK IS NO REASON TO MUTILATE AND POISON OURSELVES.

The second paradigm, a sort of "Female Paradigm" that cancer is a degenerative disease, held by the "alternative" community, seemed to make more sense. This paradigm recognizes that cancer cells are not foreign, bug-like invaders, but the body's own cells. Because the immune system is depressed, it cannot do its usual job of destroying these aberrant cells. The treatment, then, consisted of detoxifying the body and building the immune system back up to health by restoring the strength of the healing systems. When the vitality of the body is restored through positive, *supportive* methods such as nutrition, rest, group therapy, exercise, vitamins, water therapy, juice detoxification, visualization, meditation, laughter, spiritual activity, and love, the stage will be set for the healing mechanisms to be set

---

[14] Love, Susan, M.D., *Dr. Susan Love's Breast Book.* Reading, Mass. Addison-Wesley. 1990. p. 377.

in motion. The foundation has been built for the body to do the tremendous job of restoration and self-healing.

This paradigm seemed much more logical to me. It held the ring of truth. However, treatment in accordance with this view, in our free country, the United States of America, is supressed, declared illegal and is labeled "suspect" and "unproven." In some states, as the one I currently lived in, California, physicians are restricted by law from offering alternative treatments for cancer!

Funding for studies on alternative treatments does not seem to be available. In fact alternative treatments do not seem to be available in this country. In Europe alternative medicine has more general acceptance. For instance, in Germany, Johanna Budwig works with flax seed oil to help her patients heal cancer.

Breast cancer research funds are low in general. A scientist would not find research into breast cancer as attractive as AIDS research, for instance, which is well-funded. Alternative research and prevention programs such as a recent proposal to put women on a low-fat diet was at first turned down for funding. It has since been reinstated, perhaps partly because of noise we women have made! Dr. Susan Love, director of the Breast Center at the University of California at Los Angeles, is one of the leaders in this progress. She says, "We have to change the direction and really put our emphasis on basic science and prevention and not such a large emphasis on treatment." ("Science" Jan. 29, 1993).

The Cancer Control Society in Los Angeles, California[15] offers information on alternative clinics which, because they offer illegal substances such as Vitamin B17 (Laetrile), have had to set up their clinics in Mexico. They will send a list of people who have gone through alternative cancer treatment and rid themselves of their cancer. Clinics in the United States offering Laetrile in the form of ground-up apricot pits have been closed down by Federal Agents in a "witch-hunt" designed to protect the medical establishment and their sale of drugs and surgery. It's important to check out alternative clinics and remedies carefully, however, as no "cure" for cancer exists.

Ralph W. Moss (no relation to myself) does a fine job in his book *The Cancer Industry* in showing that the war on cancer was really a war to promote the sales of chemotherapy drugs and supress natural substances being used in cancer treatment. He shows how "In the name of orthodoxy, both new and traditional scientific theories are suppressed, medical records seized, clinics shut down, and innovative clinicians thrown in jail." He explains how the American Cancer Society maintains a black list on unconventional methods that is worthy of the Inquisition.

He tells us of the economic incentive to "sell" mammo-

---

[15] Cancer Control Society, 2034 Berendo Street, Los Angeles, California 90027.

grams as regular routine examinations even though women may **get** breast cancer from these X-rays. Although mammograms may sometimes result in very early detection, widespread use of this procedure in the eighties has not resulted in lower mortality rate which has remained steady at twenty-seven per one-hundred-thousand for decades. Physicians stopped doing yearly chest X-rays when they found they caused lung cancer. It is interesting to note that men are not subjected to yearly X-rays for prostrate cancer (Prostogram). Also no incisional biopsy is used on men's genital organs because scientists took the time to develop an accurate blood test (PSA)!*

Diane Sawyer, on "Prime-Time," a television commentary show, in an undercover investigation, pointed out that mammograms are also highly inaccurate due to untrained technicians, faulty machines, blurred X-rays, and mistaken readings by radiologists of these poor-quality scans.

Moss points out the economic incentive for American surgeons to perform almost a million cancer operations each year; seventy percent of those patients also supply revenue for X-ray technicians and radiation treatment. Big business is also found in the hundreds of millions spent on chemotherapy drugs annually. The drug companies are one of the U.S.'s largest businesses. Cancer is truly an industry.

Further, insurance companies will pay for orthodox treatments only: surgery, radiation and chemotherapy, not

*I believe the AMAS blood test will replace mammograms in the future.

for "experimental" treatments. (Bone-marrow transplants, called "experimental" are an extension of the orthodox method, only using extraordinarily higher doses of cytoxic chemotherapy). He who pays the piper calls the tune.

John Wayne, as a cancer patient, subjected himself as a "guinea pig" to some of these medical treatments. His comment, before he died, to his son Michael is shot straight from the hip, "Maybe it will work for some other poor bastard!"

These orthodox treatments are often a dismal failure. They do not always cure cancer. They sometimes are helpful in cases that are caught early and increase the probability, while not offering a cure, that the patient will live for five more years. More than half of those treated will not live on for five years. About a third of the women who receive it do respond to the medical treatment and live on to an old age. That some women actually live through **both** the disease and the treatment which involves so much mutilation and poisoning is the miracle. According to alternative theories, surgery sometimes works because some of the toxic load is taken off the liver. The body can then cope with whatever toxicity is left. Do these women live *in spite of* these treatments? What else did they change in their lives? Did these women also lose weight or solve emotional problems as two women I talked to did? Perhaps the sacrifice of their breast was so traumatic they were forced to confront other issues in their lives they had up to that time avoided. And if they didn't confront those other issues or change their life, then did their cancer become systemic and begin to metastasize to other parts of their bodies? Or is cancer actually a systemic disease never "confined" to only one part of the body? Was it never a "localized" disease? Was this theory only convenient to rationalize surgery, to vindicate the amputation of the breast as being "helpful," as "saving our lives?" Dr. Susan Love agrees. In a lecture given at University of California at Los Angeles, she said she believes that breast cancer is a systemic disease which has developed over a long period of time: ten years or more. She believes "early detection" is a myth. By the time a tumor is found, the disease is perhaps ten years into its development. Cancer can get in the bloodstream by year two.

I could not see the justification for these brutal treatments. Was the 'War on Cancer' as stated by Linus Pauling, an advocate of using Vitamin C to restore health in cancer patients, "largely a fraud?"

Taxol, a new medical treatment derived from the bark of the Yew tree, may be a step in the right direction as it is derived from natural sources. However, it takes so many trees to make up the medication that environmentalists are up in arms fearing the tree's extinction. Since the treatment seems to work well for some cancer patients the medical establishment is nervous about having to phase out its economic structure based on chemotherapy and radiation.

It is promising, though very expensive. Perhaps its name was originally derived from an economic idea (tax all).

Meanwhile, there are less expensive ways to get well.

One "alternative" treatment survivor in the United States is Ann Wigmore who founded the Hippocrates Health Institute in Boston and West Palm Beach Florida. An immigrant of war-torn Europe, she found herself in the U.S. struggling with various diseases. She threw out her American diet and began treating herself with wheatgrass juice, sprouts, and a diet of raw fruits and vegetables. She currently treats cancer patients at her institute with this diet, exercise, and positive attitudes. Her book, *Be Your Own Doctor* is a fascinating account of her struggles, her treatments, and her philosophies on regaining and maintaining health.

She says, "In my work at the Hippocrates Health Institute, I have utilized the discoveries of science for over thirty years. We know that no known disease can penetrate the strength of a healthy body. A low protein, low starch, low fat and high enzyme (wheatgrass), high vitamin, highly alkaline and high mineral diet is the key. Anyone can restore health by way of detoxification and rebuilding healthy cells so that the body can heal itself. Sickness is only a failure to understand the balance of body, mind, and spirit which creates well being." (p.7)

Eydie Mae Hundsberger wrote a book about her treatment, *Eydie Mae, How I Conquered Breast Cancer Naturally.* We must admire Ann Wigmore for coming up with a substance the AMA or the FDA could not find a reason to ban or declare illegal—wheatgrass.

As for Laetrile, Ralph Moss reports: "The Hunzakuts, who live in a kingdom near Pakistan have often been reported to be virtually free of cancer. It is well established that apricots and apricot kernels form a staple in their diet unparalleled in the rest of the world." (Leaf and Launois, 1975; Renee Taylor 1960). P. 139.

Max Gerson was well known as an alternative practitioner in this country. He would take patients given up by the medical establishment and sent home to die. Often they would come into his clinic on stretchers. He would detoxify their bodies with freshly made vegetable juices throughout the day. He also employed coffee enemas to detoxify the body. These patients would "miraculously" get well. His book, *A Cancer Therapy: Results of Fifty Cases,* documents his work with patients who did not die. These people actually got well and were asymptomatic years later performing their daily activities. His clinic in Mexico now run by his daughter Charlotte, uses his detoxification methods.

On the other hand, I could see nutrition was not the entire answer. Other factors were involved in cancer. Other issues in one's life had to be confronted. Other changes had to occur. Simply relying on nutrition was not going to work either.

This was graphically illustrated to me when I called Santa Monica Imaging Center. I was told of a case handled by Dr. Porrath's office.

A woman named Sharon, in her mid-thirties, with a husband and two children, came into the office with a breast lump. After a mammogram indicated she might have cancer, she refused a biopsy or any medical treatment and instead went to Mexico to a clinic for Laetrile treatments. When she returned to the United States the doctor was amazed to see her tumor had regressed, shrunk to a very small size.

However, after returning home, even though she continued to take the Laetrile, after a few months her tumor mushroomed in size. Her breast became ulcerated as the cancer ate through the skin. She then took her doctor's advice and submitted to a mastectomy. Three or four months after surgery, she died.

Of course, I did not have adequate information about Sharon. The fact was that Laetrile helped in tumor regression while she was away from home in Mexico. However, Laetrile did not work when she later returned to her home situation.

The blatant fact that came out of this all was that neither nutrition alone, even Laetrile, was enough to instigate permanent tumor regression. That surgery did not prevent death from breast cancer at an advanced stage was also sharply illustrated by this case. I knew that in devising my own program I could not rely on diet or diet supplements alone. There are many other factors in a woman's life that can cause illness. The fact that Laetrile helped this woman when she was on "vacation" but not at home suggested to me other problems in her environment, perhaps psychological. What stresses and emotional problems contributed to Sharon's illness that she experienced a respite from when she was in Mexico?

Confronted with this information, I knew that I needed to devise a program that would cover *all the bases*. Diet would be only one part.

I had by now decided to devise my own health program and stare the tumors and possible cancer down in the strongest attempt I could muster. When confronted with illness, one goes to the doctor. I had gone to my doctor not feeling ill. But he had found evidence in the form of two tumors that I was, in fact, very ill. I might be on the brink of death.

I came to the realization I could no longer rely solely on my doctor. Yes, he was still my partner in health. But as he was now screaming at me to see a surgeon, he now had to become a "silent partner." He had made it clear to me that aware of it or not, I was becoming seriously and chronically ill. He had set a deadline, postponing catastrophe, the possible surgical removal of my breast and/or a hysterectomy. It was extremely important to me for several reasons to keep my breast intact. As a single woman, I feel I need my breasts to attract males. As well as sexual attraction, the breasts are an important part of love play. Amputation would mean humiliation and victimization. Women who have hysterectomies often lose their sex drive; they are "castrated." I was not willing to go through such extreme sacrifices of the integrity of my femininity and self-esteem. I did not believe, at any rate, that these drastic measures would work to save my life or stop the spread of disease.

Slowly evolving into my blurred consciousness as I tried to wrestle down my fears, was the idea of constructing a comprehensive health program covering all aspects of my life. The idea that I could take full responsibility for my own health without relying on my doctor *or* any alternative clinic, without leaving home, without paying out huge sums of money which I did not have was appealing. Without any help but my own willpower and ingenuity, readings, and friends' encouragement, **I would get well.**

It seemed that the two paradigms, one of which suggested treatments that tore the body down; the other—unofficial—that built the body up had various reasons for coming into being. The heavily economic rationale for the Termite theory of breast cancer led me to distrust and throw out this concept and approach entirely. Kimberly's case showed this paradigm was fallacious. Her experience had showed me the medical treatment led to dehumanization, defeminization, mutilation, and the general wreckage of the human body. For all her sacrifice, there was no cure. Kimberly still had cancer, only now it was *lung* cancer. I saw complete and utter devastation along with her disease. I could hardly bear the news that she had decided to continue with the same medical treatment that she had *not responded to*. She told me she was happy with her doctor and the care she was being given. She had decided to continue with the "traditional" treatments. "Everyone has to get well her own way," she told me.

Cancer seemed intimately tied up with the personality. Outlook and attitude seemed important. The question I found myself asking was, "Did Kimberly want to live or die?" This is the same question I wound up asking myself.

Although I have never been very fond of using myself as a human guinea pig, I could see no other alternative.

What choices did I have?

Number one: I could ignore the lumps. That wouldn't work. I already knew I had two lumps. Dr. Furr had found them. The lump in my breast was palpable; it felt like a stone. The lump in my uterus was causing a painful backache as it grew and pressed against my internal organs. I was aware of these lumps at all times. If they were malignant, I might subsequently die. So that option was definitely out.

Number two: I could go with the medical treatment. My body would be mutilated and disfigured, poisoned, and irradiated. I would probably never have a bank account again. My studio and home would be sold to pay for the treatments since I don't have health insurance. Even if the treatments worked, which was less than a fifty percent chance, I would be so depressed at being disfigured and losing everything, my life wouldn't seem worth living. When I considered this option, I fell into a deep well of depression. Torture just isn't "my thing."

Number three: I could create my own health plan from what I'd read and my own prior experience, go with it, believe in it, make it work. I would thus still live, keep my breasts, keep my health, and continue my life and my art.

After reviewing this list, I could see that there was really only one choice. I decided I definitely wanted to live. I did not want to subject myself to surgery. And thus I began this GREAT EXPERIMENT OF MY LIFE.

MOTEP—The Tumor Wipe-Out and Prevention Program

5

The Marathon Olympic Tumor Eradication Program (MOTEP) was devised under the gun. It is continually being refined as I have adopted it for life; but at the time I developed it, I was excruciatingly tied to a deadline. During the month that followed I was to take the voyage spiraling downward into the depths of chronic, debilitating illness. As the disease progressed, I was to become horribly, grotesquely ill. However, illness viewed as a creative challenge is much different than a passive succumbing to hopeless fear. For me, to actively battle for one's life is enormously better than leaving treatment decisions to some authority figure that one "trusts." Instead I put my trust in my own immune system and my battle plan.

I had a few but very valued helpers: Dr. Furr, who had found the lumps, set off the alarm and gave me a deadline;

Mike Cole at the YMCA who helped me devise a physical fitness and body fat percentage goal; my father, Ben Moss, an avowed health-nut and self-healer; Dr. David B. Clark, an encourager and supporter, cheering me on and giving me tips; Sandy Naito, my Japanese friend at the "Y" who taught me about the Japanese diet and health methods, and all my concerned friends who supported me.

This program may be worth a look to you. I believe it is a good prevention program. I can't guarantee it will work if you have a lump. You can try it at your own risk. But any method you try is going to be at your own risk. Even if you catch a lump early, there is no guarantee that the medical establishment's treatment will cure you of cancer. Certainly though, early or "earlier" detection is the most important factor in any treatment plan. Lumps can be caught early through regular self-breast exam and palpation yearly by a skilled gynecologist. Most of the women I interviewed for this book who had breast cancer had **negative** mammograms.

MOTEP is a lot of hard work. It is no "magic bullet." The "easy" route of going to a surgeon and letting him cut away the disease is rejected. This fund raising fantasy of the medical establishment had proven its worthlessness in front of my eyes.

I decided to take full responsibility for my health. This was the number one most important step. Without "blaming"

myself or feeling guilty, I was ready to accept full responsibility. Thus I was able to shoulder full consequences for my
treatment plan. I was putting my life on the line. This was not
a theoretical conjecture or opinion. This was my life.

I accepted full consequences for my decision, and the
fact that I might die. I chose to go my own route, to seek and
confront the basic cause of the degeneration of my body.
I believed if my program was adequate and covered all
aspects of my life, I could do the deep inner work of self-
healing. Even as I got seriously ill, I didn't wince and stop
or give up. I let my body go through what it needed to go
through. My role was to urge my body on, supporting it in
its valiant efforts to regain health. I had to be strong against
the disease, to oppose and conquer it rather than succumb
to it. I chose to believe that even if I had cancer, I could cure
myself and I could do it, or at least begin to do it, within the
time-limit of two months that Dr. Furr had given me. I had to
work fast! Here then is MOTEP:

1. Visualization, prayer, chanting. Twice a day.
2. A semi-vegetarian diet, extremely low fat, some
   fish, no dairy, few eggs.
3. Under-eating slightly (for a period of a month—
   cutting calories but not nutrients).
4. Fresh juiced carrots (about eight) every day and
   fresh juiced oranges (about four) every day.

5. One hour of vigorous exercise five or six days a week. (I chose to swim one mile per day).
6. Sauna before and after exercise.
7. Rubbing one-half fresh cut lemon on my breast lump twice a day for directly applied Vitamin C. This can be alternated with flax seed oil.
8. Eight hours sleep every night, short nap mid-day, if possible.
9. Elimination of all pills and drugs, even prescription that aren't life-essential.
10. Elimination of all caffeine and alcohol.
11. Group therapy.
12. Making it a point to help and encourage others.
13. Giving love to others and giving it to myself, generously.
14. Smiling and laughing as much as possible. (Inspired by Norman Cousins).
15. Inducing in myself a feeling of well-being no matter what my actual circumstances were.
16. Deciding no matter how much stress I was under, I was not going to take it out on my body.
17. Increase in Vitamin Supplements (A, Selenium) added to my usual B,C,E, Calcium, and Zinc. Foods containing Laetrile. (See appendix.)
18. Asking for help and support from others instead of playing loner.

19. Having absolute faith that MOTEP would eventually work and I would heal myself.
20. A strong determination to survive, will to live, and a longing to share my experience with others.

I put the spiritual aspect of my program first because it was the basis of my strength and willpower to go through this rather strenuous and disciplined program in which I would rebuild my sick body. My friend Cheri says we can stick to programs like these because I'm a fanatic like she is. She has been into holistic medicine for years.

My unwavering faith and confidence that I would eventually succeed was soon put to the extreme test. Although I implemented the program immediately, during the following month I became very alarmed at my appearance. My face took on a horrible sallow yellow-green look. I felt very fatigued. My hair lost its normal thickness and bouyancy and began to resemble a sad, wet mop. My general health slipped rather rapidly away. I began to feel I was losing the grasp on my life that had always tied me closely to my energy source. Normally, I am an early-riser, a vigorous exerciser, and hard worker. Now my joy and vigor seemed to be atrophying along with my body. Nevertheless, I stuck to my spartan regimen with all the dedication, focus, concentration and willpower I could conjure up. **I MADE MYSELF CONTINUE!**

The basis of my program was a general detoxification,

de-stressing and building up of my body. Nutritionally, I loaded my body with vitamins, freshly made juices and whole grains, as well as fruits and vegetables. I found my favorite grain to be barley. As a fiber it performed almost like a vacuum cleaner—ridding my body of extraneous cholesterol, stress hormones, and carcinogenic substances. Barley is one of the foods that contains Laetrile, a known cancer-fighting and tumor dissolving nutrient. Somehow barley seemed to induce a feeling of well-being more than other grains. Carrot juice is medicinal, especially for lumps and tumors in the body. Beta carotene is a proven tumor-fighter.

During the first month on the program my body threw out a lot of junk. It seemed as though I spent half my life in the bathroom as my body cleaned house. At times I was so gassey, I competed with the resident skunk family in my yard. My body was "taking out the garbage." I stunk.

I had a nightmare one month into MOTEP: My left breast was rotting, becoming a putrid, green mass of mouldy, sick tissue with a horrid rancid smell. This vivid dream seemed to go on the entire night. It was in technicolor and seemed horribly real as I watched my breast disintegrate. The smell was putrid and memorable. The odor coming off my breast was a powerful stench: sickening! I woke up in a cold sweat at my usual time, 5:30 A.M. I could still smell that putrid, rotten odor! Now I knew it was real; my breast was starting to rot!

I ran into the bathroom where I splashed some cold water on my face distorted with terror and sweat.

At the "Y" I discovered the bad news. My left breast had now turned a glowing neon-red color and was burning hot to the touch. It was also inflamed and as hard as a rock. I couldn't raise my left arm. It had turned into cement, stiff and swollen. The lymph nodes must now be involved. My face was now alarmingly yellow. My breast felt like it was composed of swarming, angry bees. I experienced sharp stabbing pains in my breast periodically, a knife by some unseen assailant.

I knew then that I was very ill. I might have cancer.

I had not yet read *Dr. Susan Love's Breast Book*. Nor had I gone to a surgeon who might have told me what she says on p. 269:

> "Inflammatory Breast Cancer is a special kind of advanced breast cancer and it's a serious one. Fortunately, it's also rare—it only accounts for one to four percent of all breast cancers. It's called inflammatory because its first symptoms are usually a redness and warmth in the skin of the breast without a distinct lump.
>
> "With inflammatory breast cancer, you have cancer cells in the lymph vessels of your skin, which is what makes the skin red, the cancer is blocking the drainage of fluid from the skin.

"Statistics in the past suggested that most women with this aggressive cancer had a survival rate of about 18 months with two percent surviving five years."

Inflammatory carcinoma is often diagnosed without a biopsy. Jane Cowles, in her book, *Informed Consent,* states:

"Inflammatory carcinoma is a rare and deadly disease considered by some doctors to be diagnosed solely on clinical evidence specifically diffuse swelling, firmness, and redness of the skin and breast."[16]

These symptoms were shocking and humiliating. I was embarrassed by the hideous and grotesque look of my breast and my leaded arm. Reviewing my high-risk history, and the heavy duty stress I was under at work, I realized I had almost every risk factor. Was I a time-bomb waiting to go off? At this point I looked like one!

The decision I made staring dumbly in my mirror at my shockingly ludicrous breast was that I could beat the odds. I went down to the swimming pool with a steel-willed determination and yanking my wooden arm out of the water (at times I could only use one arm) began stridently to do my laps. I was going to conquer this thing, whatever it was. I was going to get rid of the lump, the redness, the feverish condition, and the pain in the less than one month left that

---

[16] Jane Cowles, p. 188.

I had to go. I was not going to submit myself to mutilation and poisoning. Nor would I be victimized into financial ruin by the medical establishment or vanquished by some ridiculous disease! I refused to be intimidated by the gaudy display, this circus manifesto of my very sick breast.

What I didn't know then is that the reaction was a "flare-up" my body needed to kill the cancer cells. This bodily induced fever creates the sauna-like conditions to obliterate the cancer, just as a fever kills viruses in a case of the flu. The subsequent bee-hive of activity as cells, the cytokines (cells that move), which rushed around in my breast was also part of the healing process. I had detoxified my body to the point that it was able to go through this necessary reaction. I was to find out about all this later from reading Dr. Max Gerson's writings and new research into healing processes. For instance, temperature significantly affects the immune system. When microorganisms or mutated cells invade the body, the immune system is stimulated to produce chemical substances called pyrogens, one form of cytokine. These stimulate the hypothalamus in the brain, the seat of temperature changes, to raise the "set point" or thermostat so the body can create a very hot temperature, or fever. The body then "sterilizes" these invaders out. A recent discovery, according to Dr. David Clark, is "heat-shock proteins." These proteins wrap around normal cells during a fever, protecting them. Perhaps that is why only my left breast got firey hot, while the rest of my body stayed the normal temperature.

Unfortunately, Dr. Gerson, though a pioneer and a genius-level alternative healer, had never been able to have his views and discoveries widely accepted. The economic politics of cancer had kept his findings from the light of public knowledge, insuring that the disfiguring and toxic "treatments" I had seen Kimberly go through were the accepted "traditional" ones. Likewise, Dr. Kanematsu Sugiura's research at Memorial Sloan-Kettering showing that Laetrile "inhibited metastases to the lungs" was buried. Might Kimberly's breast cancer not have metastasized into her lungs if she had eaten foods such as apricot pits, which contain the vitamin B17?

It seemed a labyrinth of commercial interest and politics had led to a general ignorance of the causes and preventions of cancer and how the body reacts in its *own healing procedures.* That Kimberly's lung cancer was, in all probability preventable, made me very angry. The entire treatment process she was going through which seriously compromised her immune system while not curing her had brought fuel to my fire. I was just as ignorant and in the dark as the general public about how cancer either metastasized or was healed. I knew absolutely nothing about the healing reaction I was going through. I had no idea it *was* a healing reaction. As far as I was concerned at the time, the bizarre reaction was a part of my illness and a sign that my program "wasn't working or hadn't kicked in yet." I did not lose faith in my program. I did not give in and call my doctor to tell him I was ready to see the surgeon. I continued on my MOTEP program with the determination to see my illness through its various stages until its conclusion when I would get well. **I would will myself to live.**

SIDE EFFECTS OF MOTEP

It's only fair, since we know the horrendous side-effects of medical treatments for breast cancer that we go over the side effects of MOTEP as I experienced them.

1. An increase in vitality and energy.
2. A much better figure.
3. Loss of all bodily cellulite and other unsightly fat.
4. Hair grows back normal color instead of gray.
5. Hair has more luster and thicker texture.
6. No one can believe that you are "that old."
7. Better eyesight.
8. Lowered blood pressure.
9. Better work performance and subsequently more business success.
10. Increased popularity.
11. A completely changed, happier life.

A Typical Day on the MOTEP Program

I awaken automatically at 5:30 a.m. now. It's pitch dark. Whose idea was this anyway? Remembering that I am fighting for my life, I jump out of bed. Getting up so early was a more or less good idea. I sold myself on it, so I do it. It's still hard at times even when I go to bed early.

I stumble to the bathroom to splash water on my face and start my routine which is to rub my breast with half a cut lemon or flax seed oil.

The lemon would seem to burn, but it doesn't. It is actually cooling, soothing, and refreshing. I concentrate my mind on the lump area and as I apply the lemon or oil, I incorporate visualization, seeing myself rubbing away the lump.

Next on the agenda is chanting, visualization, and prayer after throwing on some clothes and feeding the cat. As I chant the Lotus Sutra, I concentrate on sending the sound vibrations to the lump in my breast. There is a mystical power which comes from harnessing spiritual energy that seemingly cleanses the body. A purity of feeling and calmness pierces the tangled clamor of my anxious cells, putting them to rest. The endorphins from my brain seem to kick in as an opiate, putting me in a semi-hypnotic state tuning out stressful thoughts and anxiety-filled reactions. As I sit in front of my Gohonzon (a Japanese shrine with candles and fruit), I chant Daimoku, Nam-Myoho-Renge-Kyo (loosely translated: the mystic law of cause and effect through sound vibration), over and over until I enter a trance-like state. In a semi-hypnotic state the subconscious becomes highly suggestible. This might also be achieved in other ways, for instance, through prayers, religious chants, or incantations. Spiritual rituals have a life-affirming quality. They seem to tap into the subconscious mind creating a positive mental affirmation. I can feel "all knowing," connecting to the universe, and feeling that I am headed into the direction of health. I continue to aim this sound vibration to the lump in my breast. Also, I chant for others: this morning, I chant for Kimberly, whose lungs are now filled with cancer cells. Despite the turmoil in the world (the war in the Middle-East is being fought) and the stresses in my life and the lives of my friends, I finally achieve a feeling of peace and serenity as I chant through the turmoil I feel. I chant hard like a lion throwing out the roar of healing energy. Pent-up repressed energy and anger can be thrown out of the soul this way. Repressed anger is suspected as a culprit in tumors and cancer. The cancer personality has trouble with or *cannot express anger.* They may repress negative feelings in fear of alienating others if they "leak out" and they may lose their friendship. This anger and frustration is held within the body eating away its vitality. Chanting gets out these tensions. There is a wonderful peace which fills the mind, soul, and spirit creating a powerful feeling of well-being. I have not found this sort of incredible sensation of peace any other way. It fills my agitated body, calming and soothing it. I feel at rest, at peace, at home.

After chanting I do a bit of studying. I read Vice President Tsuji's guidance in the Sept. 1987 "Seikyo Times," a Buddhist publication:

"Although you may see it manifested in the light bulb, the law of electricity does not enable you to overcome disease. It does not enable you to calm hysterics and for most problems, it will not give you a solution. But if you know the law of life, or if you have something that embodies the law of life, you will be able to overcome disease and you will be able to change your karma."

Nichiren Daishonin, who originated the form of Buddhism I practice, writes: "Nam-Myoho-Renge-Kyo is the roar of the lion. What disease can therefore be an obstacle?"

And Daisaku Ikeda writes: "Healing is a restoration to the whole. The words 'healing,' 'whole,' and 'holy' all derive from the same root. Holy is being complete, being connected as a person and with other persons, being connected to the planet. Pain is a signal that the part is separate from the whole. This observation is not limited to physiological pain—but it can be applied to all that ails our contemporary civilization. Human wholeness refers to that vibrant state of being in which embracing history and tradition, we can absorb and embody the rhythms of universal life in new patterns of action and activity. The experience of human wholeness is one of deep fulfillment and enables us to manifest qualities such as composure, generosity, tolerance, and consideration."

Driving to the "Y" in the dark, the stillness and peace of the environment, the universe, is a continuation of this feeling. That is until I get to the locker room where there is a TV. The Persian Gulf war seems ironically timed. I must eliminate anxiety and exude calmness in order to get well. The world is not cooperating. Norman Cousins recommends comedy shows like "Candid Camera." But the camera is now pointed at a blonde steel-jawed reporter who looks frightened out of his mind. He is enshrouded by the night sky ablaze periodically with streaks of yellow and scud-missile lights. Later he is captured and thrown into a prisoner-of-war compound. There is no comedy on any station. Fear and anxiety and destruction have invaded all the networks. Just as Marilyn Monroe predicted, war has become entertainment.

I wrest myself from the TV. This reporter is wiring my nerves even more than they already are re-wired with recession, unrequitted love, and breast-lump disease.

I've decided to concentrate on swimming during my tumor eradication program; my goal is to swim one mile every morning until I reach full health. Sandy, my Japanese friend, is in the locker room already, another very early riser.

Today we talk about the Japanese diet as the women there have the lowest rate of breast cancer. She tells me they eat dried fish and miso soup with seaweed for breakfast; noodles such as buckwheat for lunch, and fresh fish and vegetables with rice for dinner. No dessert is served unless it is fresh fruit or gelatin. I think of ways to trim down my diet further. Could I ever achieve that sort of sparsity? At this point, I'm willing to try anything that would work.

Now for a sauna. It's very hot and dry as I lie down feeling the intense heat. I perform my three-step breast exam. The lump is definitely still present and accounted for, hard as a rock. My breast feels like barbed-wire jello. The rock-tumor-lump is granite, so permanent and solid. How can I chisel it down? I try closing my eyes and visualizing the lump as a frozen piece of butter which melts under the intense, dry sauna heat. Doing my mental part of the exam, I feel a pinching at the spot where the lump is located. I visualize a large pair of pliers and "tweeze" out the lump with this tool.

I shower off the sweat and head for the pool. The heater is broken. Nevertheless, I ease into the chilly water wondering again whose idea this actually is. As I swim, I hum, something the lifeguard comments laughingly about. I again use this sound vibration to shatter the lump, directing the music straight to it. I also use a white light which I visualize, like a laser beam shooting it to my breast-rock. I watch it detonate as if hit by a scud missile, into thousands of minute pieces.

I watch as these pieces float away into the water.

A mile is a long way. At first I still feel "uptight." My body is in an ultra-stressed-out condition. I feel it is necessary to visualize a very large hypodermic needle with a gigantic loading tube labeled "WELL BEING" in big block letters. I give myself an imaginary shot. I feel the pinch as the needle enters my arm. Suddenly, I relax. This allows me to be able to swim peacefully through the soothing water. After almost a full hour of swimming, I am no longer tense. My body feels alive and flexible. I'm ready to conquer the day.

Another sauna is taken to warm up. I visualize my lump relaxing into space and disappearing like a ghost never to return. Then after a shower, I get back into my work clothes. I walk out of the "Y" refreshed, rejuvenated, and relaxed. I feel confident that I have made more inroads against my disease. Enough of these daily energetic reversals and I **will** be well.

I get the newspaper and look at pictures of more scud missiles, frightened Generals, a pale President, and a mean dictator. I try to separate what's happening "out there" from what's going on inside myself. I repeat my determination to stay relaxed, creating an "invisible shield" which protects myself physically from my own stresses and world events and allows me to remain at peace. It's hard.

At home again, I make a simple breakfast of fresh-squeezed orange juice, and a natural granola with no preservatives, fresh fruit, and herb tea. I pack a lunch of half a sandwich on whole-grain bread with a filling of vegetables and three or four kinds of fruit: unsprayed New Zealand apples, a mango, red grapes, apricots, or peaches, whatever is in season. I concentrate on orange and red-colored fruits that have lots of beta carotene.

At work I face my large canvas, "Night Sky," in my beautiful skylit studio. I am struggling with it, slashing at it. It is going through its usual ugly stage, wet, and greasy looking. It will finally dry to a wonderful, satin sheen. I wrestle with it all day. It seems to go well; then it eludes me. Painting is a mystery and a contest with myself. One that never stops frustrating and thrilling me. I am caught up in the drama of an intense war painting with its deep indigo blues and scud missile yellow-white areas of moonlight and explosion. I am attempting an intensely spiritual experience. This is a war painting that I am dedicating to the P.O.W.'s.

The studio is quiet. A few friends call but because of the recession, business has ground to a halt. A very nice couple want to buy the study for "Night Sky" but change their mind because of the war and the recession. They say they "love my work" but this, unfortunately, does not pay my bills. I decide just to separate this financial anxiety from my physical life. I've never gone completely broke during my painting career, though once I got down to a total of two hundred dollars in the bank. Something always happens.

Finally the work speaks and someone can't resist buying it. The painting goes straight-forward, but the business is a roller coaster; feast or famine as my freind, Craig Kauffman, says. He's been in the "business" longer and is more successful than I. But he's older and this is a "long-haul" proposition. Most people get nowhere in this terribly hard field. I feel fortunate to be able to earn my livelihood doing what I love to do—painting and drawing. Shows in New York, Chicago, San Francisco, Los Angeles, La Jolla, and Washington, D.C. have helped. Hundreds of collectors have enabled me to continue my life's work.

At noon I stop, exhausted from the outpouring of emotion vested in executing "Night Sky." I eat my vegetarian lunch and drink mineral water, then I take a short half-hour nap. I wait for the mail person. Perhaps one of my galleries has sold or rented some work for me and I will receive a check that will allow me to keep painting.

At one o'clock, I automatically wake up. This system has somehow been set up in my brain to work. I always have more energy in the afternoon this way. I go back to "Night Sky" for another four hours of battle. This painting is taking seemingly forever; I end up working for months before it finally winds to a conclusion.

At five, I quit. Having expended all my energy, heart, soul, creative powers, and experience on one work, I am ready to stop. This type of self-discipline, to work all day without a "whistle," timeclock, or pay check is something I naturally do. It doesn't seem out-of-the-ordinary for me. I've been doing it for over twenty years. It is now routine.

At home, more war news on TV. Why aren't there the comedy shows Norman Cousins watched to get well? All the humor and positive emotions have been pre-empted by the horror of war.

I juice about eight large carrots (the very largest ones have the most beta carotene) and drink the delicious tumor fighter. I then fix a simple dinner of whole grains and vegetables. Tonight, it's pearl barley (containing Laetrile), a comforting high-fiber, low-fat food. Vegetables and a tomato juice sauce (more beta carotene) completes the dish. The grain is accompanied by a big raw vegetable salad with the darkest leafed lettuce I can find, onions, and raw garlic (selenium), tomatoes, cabbage (cruciferous vegetable, a known tumor fighter), and some sunflower seeds for protein. A dressing of olive oil, flax-seed oil, balsamic vinegar, and cracked pepper and I have a satisfying dinner that will also be extremely low fat and full of tumor-fighting nutrients. For dessert, I have dates (lots of Vitamin A) or other fresh fruit and herb tea.

After dinner I talk to a few friends on the phone, call collectors to ask them to visit the studio, write in my diary, and chant. Calming any anxiety, the chanting again is directed to the lump. Visualization is used to "see" the sound vibration disintegrating the lump into a million, zillion pieces. In a trance-like state, I create my own reality, one in which I am well and successful, my breast clean, and my bank account full.

I try to get to bed early, before ten. I now realize I am fighting for my life.

Seven days before my appointment, the lump is still depressingly present. What will happen to me? I decide to have an all-encompassing faith that the program is working. *I will put complete trust in my body.* I continue steadfastly on my routine. Against all odds this program is going to work and it *will* work on schedule. I feel generally better and my face is no longer the horrid yellow color I get when I am extremely ill. I am less terrified, also; the calm feeling, "high life-condition," peace-of-mind, and feeling of well-being that I have worked so hard to try to induce in myself seems to be breaking through. I feel, somehow, *victorious*, though nothing has physically changed. The lump is still there, hasn't budged or changed during my monthly cycle. But something is different. I have a premonition I've turned the fork of the road back to health.

Five days before my appointment, I do my self-breast exam in the sauna as usual. **There is no lump.** I can't believe it! It's astonishing. I planned this miracle, but when it comes down to the bottom-line, did I really think it was going to work? I do the exam again, and then again. In doing the mental portion, I can tell my breast is still not normal. The barbed cells are still swarming around, but now there is no pinched feeling where the lump was. My first thought—there is no lump and I still have five days to go! I am ecstatic. During my swim that morning my breast began to itch like crazy as a wound does when it is healing.

After the totally euphoric, victorious wave of emotion sweeps over me, I lurch back to a stern state of mind. I realize I have to continue working to keep the tumor away. This I manage to do keeping up the MOTEP program. I now decide I have to follow the program the *rest of my life.* My body learned how to create a breast and uterine lump, perhaps cancer. Now I have taught it, or helped it, to heal and discard the tumors. I have a Greater Knowledge now of how my body works. I have been through a sort of spiritual growth, a lesson in extreme self-control. I have found keys to my own health through discipline. This low fat diet, under eating, chanting, prayer, visualization, group therapy, high-energy exercise, and self-induced ''well-being'' came together to produce a miracle. And right on schedule! Dr. Furr is in for a surprise.

Five days later I drive to Dr. Furr's office. It's mid-afternoon and the office is deadly quiet. EVERYONE KNOWS. The place has the feel of a funeral parlor. I am the only happy, confident person in the place.

Dr. Furr rushes me into the office, a stern, angry look on

his face. He is ready to order me over to the surgeon, straight-jacketing me if necessary. This is an emergency case!

I sit calmly and tell him, I think I got rid of it. But I let him know its up to him to decide.

He nods sharply, looking very skeptical at this report.

He has me lie on the table. Using his full weight he practically jumps as he performs the breast exam with all the pressure of his hands he can muster. But he can't find a lump. He remembers exactly where it was. "It was right here?" he states, a perplexed look coming into his face. He tries the other breast to no avail. He goes back to the left breast and tries two more times.

I can't help saying, "I challenge you to find the lump."

But try as he might, he can't find it.

Finally exhausted, with a weak smile, he gives in. He concedes a victory to me.

"How did you do it?" he demands weakly.

I briefly outline my MOTEP program.

He offers to show a video-tape of my program in his office if I care to make one. He admits he is a vegetarian. NOW he tells me! He offers to learn Buddhism! I have never seen Dr. Furr this talkative. This interested. What is my secret? He's like a recent convert ready to join my "Church of Health."

Everyone in the office seems jubilant as he says with joy in his voice, "See you next year!!"

It's a huge, momentous victory. Everyone in the office

feels it. But I know I still have work to do. My breast still hurts; I am not yet back to normal. Nor will I be for seven more months of continuous, relentless work.

But the major crisis is past. I'm back on the road to health. And I have a plan now to get fully well and stay well. The Great Secret of ridding the body of tumors is simply to de-toxify and de-stress the body. In supporting the body in all positive health-giving ways, self-healing will soon take place. One becomes a cheerleader, a bystander, watching the miraculous ''cure'' take place.

As for Dr. Furr, after reading this manuscript he decided not to take any chances with his own health and joined the ''Y'' himself. When I see him every morning he still has that look of astonishment on his face!

Diedre Morgan— A Designing Woman Who Designed Away Her Breast Cancer 6

Diedre Morgan is a vivacious, elegant woman in her fifties whom I met when I walked into a spacious blue-chip art gallery, newly installed in Beverly Hills. She works there as a gallery assistant.

We immediately hit it off. I told my friends that I felt an immediate spiritual connection with her.

After visiting the gallery several times and having her over to look at my work at the studio, we became friends. I mentioned my experience in self-lumpectomy which I planned to write about. To my amazement she said the very same thing had happened to her. She agreed to share her story.

When she was forty-two, she had gone to her gynecologist for her regular yearly exam. He had found a lump in her breast. He told her this lump was not something to ignore and instructed her to get a mammogram.

"At the time I was way too busy to stop or interrupt my schedule," she told me her hands waving in the air. "I was a designer of maternity clothes and a trip to Saks Fifth Avenue in New York couldn't be postponed."

She did, however, get a mammogram which proved the doctor correct in his findings. The lump looked seriously threatening. The next day the doctor called and ordered her to see a surgeon.

"I told my doctor that I would call him in a week when I returned from my business trip."

However, in New York, the trip became lengthened. "My mother, who lives back East, became ill with gall-bladder cancer and I felt an obligation to stay for a month and take care of her while she went into the hospital for surgery." Her eyes got very wide as she exclaimed, "My doctor was *frantic* and called me everyday. He told me to get back here. I had to see a surgeon. NOW!"

I told him, "I do self-healing."

Diedre went to Cape Cod to take care of her mother. While there she would implement her self-healing program. This is how she describes it:

"Every morning I would stay in bed and do visualization, after awakening, for twenty to thirty minutes. First I would focus on the third eye, the eye in the middle of my forehead and think about and "see" a white light emanating from this eye. I would pull down this white light letting it go throughout my body and circle it through my breast until I attained a peaceful, clean state."

She would perform this "white light" spiritual cleansing once a day only. Along with this spiritual exercise, she supplemented and changed her normally vegetarian diet ("I haven't eaten meat in twenty years except for once or twice a year at a party," she explains) only by eliminating all caffeine and taking more Vitamin A and E. "I took maybe three Vitamin A pills a day."

She noted that although the vitamins helped strengthen her, the healing "wasn't external." She sees her healing as an entirely internal process and explains, "Find a wavelength and work with it. Accept it as a healing source."

Then quietly, "There is a lot of motivation in breast cancer. I had to get rid of it."

Diedre believes we look to diet and exercise because we are physical people, but the "truth is if we were really evolved enough, if we really believed, we would be able to use our spiritual strength to cure ourselves of anything."

"We need faith and trust in our own abilities to heal. We give power to diet. Diet has nothing to do with it. We want to put "healing power" in a bottle. But what we really must do is empower ouselves. Get us to be true to ourselves and to believe we can self-heal. The power to heal our own bodies is within ourselves."

I asked Diedre if she had been under stress before the doctor found her breast lump.

"Tremendous stress," she said, "During the last three or four years there was enough stress to put me in a mental hospital. "She explained how tough her design business had been. She saw herself as "out of sync" in a state of frustration, anger, and resentment. She believes her lump evolved out of her flailing emotions and frustrations. To rid herself of the cancer she had to turn her emotional state around. To calm herself and cleanse herself of ugly turmoil was her foremost goal.

"Do you think helping your mother aided your own healing?" I asked. I recalled to her the night I had visited my Buddhist friend Jeanne Hall. She had been rushed to the hospital after an abcess was lanced causing blood poisoning throughout her body. I brought her pumpkin bread. We joked about the plastic pudding the hospital served which she didn't have to eat as I had brought a healthier substitute dessert. Although she looked very weak and tired, wired up to the intravenous tubes which fed her antibiotics to combat the poisoning, we chanted together, doing evening gongyo. This praying together was really wonderful, a healing experience for me, though it was Jeanne who was supposedly the sick one. I was in the middle of my own fight for my health, though I didn't look as ill. Nor were there any tubes hooked up to my arms. As I left the hospital after helping Jeanne, I felt a healing energy stronger, much more forceful, than I had experienced chanting alone.

Diedre considered this theory. She said she "recognized the spiritual law" that I had described and thought there was a counterpart in helping others to heal thus creating healing energy for oneself.

She repeated the main goal of self-healing was to empower ourselves, to get us to be true to ourselves, and to *believe* absolutely in our own curative powers.

She never did any self-breast exams. During the month she was away, she concentrated on healing herself and helping her mother without worrying at all whether the lump was still there or not. This impressed me. I had anxiously done my self-breast exam everyday during my program. She said she hadn't bothered herself with any self-examinations.

"I had an obstruction," she said. "That was what I had to get rid of."

She returned home a month later, on a Monday, having gotten her mother through her catastrophe successfully. On Tuesday her doctor called and set up an appointment for her with a surgeon for Wednesday.

The surgeon set up the X-rays from the mammogram and began the breast-exam. He performed the manual procedure once, got a puzzled look on his face, and went back to X-rays. After three times of this round-about procedure, he gave in.

"X-rays don't lie," he said. "But you have nothing. I don't know what you did, but whatever it was, I suggest that you keep it up."

That was ten years ago. Diedre has had no recurrence. She now does healing work with others. She feels that the right breast is connected to external events. Problems with it mean you are out-of-sync and filled with frustration, anger, and resentment. The left breast is more atuned to female emotions, problems with love. The emotions of hostility and great anger which a woman might turn onto herself might trigger a lump. There is, she feels, a definite trigger mechanism.

"You do it to yourself," she explains.

She feels physical symptoms are easier to treat than the SOURCE OF CANCER. However, treating the physical symptoms won't always work. The mental and emotional core for the source has to be dealt with. Otherwise, despite any physical treatment, the cancer will spread.

The psyche has to undo the process. You have to work backwards. What caused the lump? What emotional problems, what frustrations with the outer world were transferred internally? What was the anger or reactive emotion that triggered the problem?

"Your psyche has to do the work which takes time and discipline and extreme focus. You have to be extremely positive. If you feel hopeless and don't want to live, how can you activate the healing process? If you feel powerless, the cancer will take over. You have to believe."

After interviewing Diedre, I had to think back on how I "did it to myself." Tensing and stressing my own body with my fears, anxieties, and emotional pain for a year before any lumps showed up seemed to be my main contribution. I had gone on a "meat kick" to somehow compensate for my problems by eating. My exercise program had degenerated into sitting in the hot whirlpool at the gym because life had not seemed worth the effort of putting out any energy to exercise. I was beyond feeling sorry for myself. Loss of hope had turned into a kind of apathy about going on with my life. Any feelings had turned inward, eating away at me, as I washed in gray despair and self-pity. Meanwhile, I ignored my plight. Maybe problems would just "go away." I stressed my body, abused my body, and ignored my body. Nothing really seemed worthwhile, anymore, so why bother? My life seemed to have reached a dead end.

When Dr. Furr discovered the signs of impending illness, a wake-up call was issued that dislodged me from my apathy and disassociation with reality. Maybe there is a reason for this illness, I thought. It's nature's alarm clock. It's time to re-examine my reasons for living. And most of all it's time to change. It's time to really take care of myself and to *really care about myself.*

Diedre Morgan realized this too. She is a living, vibrant

example of how self-healing has worked. Without disfiguring surgery or poisonous drugs, she brought herself, by her own will, back to health. She now uses her knowledge and experience to help others. Teaching others self-healing techniques, and giving them tools to aid themselves in their own quest for recovery is one of her specialties.

We both agreed that we are no longer afraid of breast cancer. Having been through a self-healing process, having been forced to examine how we helped create this illness ourselves, we learned how to reverse the process in a slow, methodical and disciplined, focused way. We have discovered, for ourselves, the cause and the cure. We now have earned our own ''insurance'' that we bought and paid for ourselves with no premiums other than the hard but very rewarding work of self-healing.

The Miracle Tumor Fighter Super-Drug Readily Available Inexpensively and How It Works

7

In 1978, during the battle to regain my health and eliminate a lump in my neck which I acquired from using carcinogenic plastic painting materials, I ran into a woman at a party in an artist's loft who told me this incredible story.

A friend of hers had a husband who was very ill with cancer. His doctor considered him a hopeless case, and after performing exploratory surgery and finding his internal organs inundated with cancer, sewed the incision back up without doing anything.

His wife was left ignorant as to the proceedings or the prognosis. Believing the surgeon had removed the cancerous tissue, and informed on alternative methods of healing, she devised her own plan to restore him to full strength. For six months, she juiced the largest carrots she could find, giving her husband this vital nourishment several times a day as he rested on the couch.

The terminally ill husband regained his strength. Within six months, in fact, he got well. His wife rushed back to the hospital, her gratitude overflowing, to congratulate the surgeon on this marvelously successful operation. The surgeon was dumbstruck. He had thought the woman came to him for sympathy and details of funeral arrangements.

This man went on to live many more productive years of life. When he finally did die many years later of other causes, an autopsy revealed absolutely no trace of cancer in his entire body!

Between getting well from the first lump and experiencing my breast and uterine lumps, I had stopped juicing carrots. But now I see that, for prevention, this ritual needs to be continued every evening.

How do carrots work?

Dr. David B. Clark explained the chemistry to me at one of his many impromptu science lectures given so generously to me over dinner. He is a hematologist (blood scientist) who works for the American Red Cross in the field of blood diseases, helping to invent a cure for hemophelia, and other blood-clotting disorders by factoring out of the blood various proteins that inherently do the job. Protein C, for example, is the substance that helps to break up blood clots in the body. He originally worked on this substance at Georgetown University in Washington, D.C. Blood clotting became a problem in hip surgery operations in which the blood had a tendency to clot unnecessarily around the site of the operation. 'Factor eight' and 'Factor nine' are substances within blood plasma which help the blood to clot. These proteins are fractionated out of the plasma to use as a "drug" for hemophelia patients whose blood, because it lacks clotting capabilities, can cause them to bleed to death from a minor cut or injury.

Just as there are clotting and unclotting factors in the blood, there are also anti-cancer factors. "Tumor necrosis factor" is a recent discovery, a protein that destroys tumors. This protein is presently being researched and factored out of the blood by scientists. Another substance, interleukin, is produced by the body to halt cancer. Scientists are currently experimenting with these natural substances that the body manufactures to combat cancer.

Dr. Clark who received his Ph.D. from Cornell University in Chemical Engineering would be the one person who could explain the therapeutic value of carrots. The fact that I originally met this "man of science" at a Buddhist meeting meant to me that I had a unique friend who combined the very latest in medical scientific technology with a strong belief in the ancient healing abilities of faith.

"We know the tumor fighting capabilities of Vitamin A," he explained. "However, Vitamin A in large doses is toxic, wreaking havoc with the kidney because it is fat-soluble.

However, two molecules of beta carotene, which is water-soluble, can be converted by the body into Vitamin A. In other words, there is little danger in overdosing from beta carotene. The worst thing that will happen with lots of carrot juice is that you will turn a bit orange in color."

Carrots have a long history of medicinal use. During the Middle Ages they were not eaten as food but were considered as a medicine only, used in the treatment of illnesses as diverse as snakebite, dizziness, and inflammation.

Ralph Moss describes the work of Bernard Peyrilhe (1735-1804) professor of chemistry at the Ecole Sante and professor-royal at the College of Surgery in Paris, who is remembered as the winner of a 1773 prize from the Academy of Lyon on the subject, "What is Cancer?" Peyrilhe advocated the use of carrot juice in the treatment of cancer. Carrot juice is also recommended in the Gerson diet to heal cancer.

In animal experiments first administered on a large scale by Harold W. Manner, Ph.D., chairman of the biology department at Loyola University, Chicago, emulsified Vitamin A was used to show dramatic results in mammary tumors in mice. In his book, *The Death of Cancer* he reports:

After 6-8 days an ulceration appeared at the tumor site. Within the ulceration was a puss-like fluid. An examination of this fluid revealed dead malignant cells. The tumors gradually underwent complete regression in seventy-five of the experimental animals. This represented eighty-nine percent of the total group. The remaining nine animals showed partial regression." 1978.

In follow-up studies involving five-hundred fifty mice with mammary tumors, he found that Laetrile alone had no effect, but a combination of Laetrile, Vitamin A, and enzymes was significantly more effective than just enzymes and/or Vitamin A. The triple combination produced tumor regression in thirty-eight out of fifty cases or seventy-six percent.

In the next chapter I will discuss the diet I constructed in which I carefully included foods rich in enzymes, Laetrile (which is a nutrient in twelve hundred foods besides apricot kernels), and Vitamin A. This diet helped to strengthen my immune system so it was able to slough off the tumors in my breast and uterus. I have adopted it for a lifetime to prevent recurrence.

A part of this diet is carrot juice made fresh each evening from about eight very large carrots.

Drinking the juice immediately after it is made provides a bath of Vitamin A which can wash over the cells, giving them instant ammunition against tumors. This regimen can be combined with visualization—actually "seeing" the juice strengthening and fortifying the cells. Visualization can also be used when drinking the juice by "watching" it dissolve breast lumps and tumors.

Epidemiological studies show that smokers who eat or

drink vegetables and fruits with high Vitamin A content are afforded some protection against lung cancer.

One of the latest findings by Dr. Robert Russell at Tufts University is that Vitamin A turns on the tumor-suppressor gene.

One "side effect" is shown by a recent study by the U.S. Department of Agriculture of people over sixty. Those with adequate carotene levels were more agile on tests of cognitive (thinking) ability.

Carrots are also well-known eye-sight improvers. Carotenoid, a substance in carrots as well as dark-green leafy vegetables such as spinach, can even help prevent cataracts according to a recent Harvard Medical Study. Cataracts are one of the leading causes of blindness in the U.S. This substance is an anti-oxidant which acts by protecting the lens of the eye from oxidative damage. Dr. Susan E. Harkinson studied the diets of fifty-thousand women and found a diet rich in carotenoids lowered the risk of cataracts by forty percent. ("Woman's Day" Feb. 23, 1993, "Eat Smart" by Denise Webb, PhD., R.D.).

All relevant studies I have seen point to carrot juice as a powerful "super-drug" in the war against breast cancer and other cancers. It has dynamic preventative properties.

The daily ritual of juicing and drinking carrot juice helped me save my breasts and my life.

The MOTEP Healing and Prevention Diet 8

In composing the MOTEP diet surrounded by my stacks of library books, cookbooks, and books on nutrition, I asked: what do the ancients recommend in two thousand B.C.? What does Modern Medical Science report in nineteen hundred ninety A.D.? What does the alternative community have to say? And finally, what worked for me before?

I was under the gun when I constructed this anti-cancer diet. I did not have time for a gradual transition in my eating habits. Under normal circumstances, a gradual change might consist of trying this diet one or two days a week, at first. Instead of a slow transition, I found it necessary to dive right into a diet consisting of only fruits, vegetables, legumes, nuts, seeds, and whole grains. I eliminated all meat including chicken and all dairy products. I did include lots of fish and two eggs a week.

This diet works. I'm living proof that the MOTEP diet is not a hypothetical or theoretical adventure into the world of nutrition by an enthusiastic college home-ec major or a Ph.D. in healing foods. This is a healing and prevention diet that actually works by restoring strength to a weakened immune system, lowering the fat content of the body, and immersing the body in tumor-fighting vitamins A, B17, C, E, and Selenium.

A major decision was deciding to go "cold turkey" and just stop eating meat. Large juicy loin lamb chops, fried chicken, Thanksgiving turkey, spare ribs, salami sandwiches, steaks, and beef stew are foods that I grew up eating—crave—am used to, and think of as a wonderful part of life. But now my life was too important. The will to live enabled me to give up meat.

Of course the idea of becoming a semi-vegetarian had, every once in a while, flitted across my mind. But just as quickly as it flitted in, it flitted out! My dad became a vegetarian twenty years ago and many of my friends existed and thrived on meatless diets. Since I seemed to be at some sort of cross-roads where my life depended on the choices I would make, I decided it was time to take the same path. I have never looked back. With a predominantly vegetarian diet my health returned, my energy increased, and my figure improved.

Along with meat, I gave up dairy products. Contrary to

the popularized slogan promoted by the dairy industry, we absolutely outgrow our need for milk (and cheese, cream, sour cream, butter, whipped cream, ice cream). While some people can tolerate yogurt, eighty percent of us are lactose intolerant and can't digest dairy products. They float around in our body undigested as mucous, causing allergies and blockages. Good substitutes for dairy products are tofu (soybean curd) and soy milk. Soybeans are rich in vegetable protein and calcium and contain no saturated animal fats and zero cholesterol. They also contain phytoestrogens which help regulate estrogen in the body.

As I planned this diet around the possiblity that my breast disease might possibly be cancer, I read what the ancients had to say first. The opinion that cancer is a nutritional disease is not a new off-the-wall alternative view but is actually four thousand years old! Carole Spearin McCauley reports in *Surviving Breast Cancer* that in the Charak Samhita, the classic seven-volume text of Indian Medicine, the cause of cancer appears as an "excess consumption of dairy food." A diet consisting of vegetables and whole grains was recommended to replace eating animals and animal products and fats.

Omni's *Future Medical Almanac* paradoxically goes backward in time to the Codex Ebers, an Egyptian medical papyrus dating from 1550 B.C. stating that garlic is an effective remedy for ailments including heart problems, headaches, bites, worms, and tumors. Garlic and onions, which are related in the vegetable family, contain selenium to protect themselves against bacteria and fungi. The body seems to be able to utilize selenium as a detoxifying agent.

Michio Kushi of the East-West Foundations offers the Macrobiotic Diet as a brake to the development of cancer. Cancer is viewed as a disease of excess. Primary factors contributing to breast cancer are listed as dairy products, fats and oils, white flour, and sugar. Secondary are drugs, eggs, meat, and poultry.

Kushi eliminates oil, fat, sugar, milk, Coca-Cola, and other extremely "yin" items. His diet contains more than half whole grains, one quarter vegetables, ten percent beans and sea vegetables, and five percent soup. This extremely "bland" diet even eliminates most fruits, except locally grown. He emphasizes that food must always be thoroughly chewed.

I kept in mind the *large amount of whole grains* while throwing out the idea of cutting down on fruits. I thrive on fruits from around the world. It seemed to me especially important to load down on yellow-red-brown-and-black fruits that would be rich in beta carotene. A large increase in fiber loaded grains help the body unload toxins and stress chemicals.

Protective factors in the macrobiotic diet are beans, leafy green and white vegetables, soy foods, and whole grains.

At the "Y" in the locker room there is a photo chart of 31 fruits and vegetables recommended by the American Cancer Society as contributing to the possible prevention of cancer. They include: apples, artichokes, red onions, bananas, strawberries, collard greens, papayas, lettuce, tomatoes, broccoli, oranges, potatoes, bell peppers, prunes, carrots, swiss chard, spinach, apricots, avocados, acorn squash, savoy cabbage, celery, cauliflower, and sweet potatoes.

I was already aware of the cruciferous family as being helpful as they contain indoles (cancer fighting nutrients): cabbage, brussel sprouts, broccoli, kale, and kohlrabi. Some of the foods rich in Laetrile (amygdalin) include chick peas, lentils, lima beans, mung bean sprouts, cashews, alfalfa, barley, brown rice, millet, apricot kernels, peach kernels, and almonds. (Amygdalin is from the Greek word Amygdale which means almond.) *R. Moss, p. 132.* Kernel preparations were used in Ancient China as tumor medicine. (See appendix for more foods containing Laetrile.) Apricot kernels are "Nature's Chemotherapy." However, do not take more than two to four a day. Large doses are poisonous.

Also very rich in Vitamin A are very dark, green leafy vegetables. I shopped for darker mustard greens, kale, collard greens, spinach, watercress, and red-leafed lettuce instead of iceburg. Asparagus became singled out by a

Pittsburgh dentist who used the vegetable to cure his lymph and eye cancers. Papayas contain a substance which breaks down scar tissue and tumorous growths.

"Fat is the enemy," a nurse who recently had a mastectomy told me. This is only partly true. We need some fats (see appendix for more information on fats and oils). However, a major goal was drastically lowering the fat content of my body. Although I was only five pounds overweight, my fat-to-lean ratio was way too high, almost five percent over what it should be. Unfortunately, as we grow older, our breasts change in composition, beginning when we are young with one hundred percent breast tissue, then half fat when we are thirty to forty years old and finally—gradually as we age and lose breast tissue—to all fat! This how we became a mature female in the first place—by adding fat. Now, however, when we grow older, this combination of more and more fat, the accumulation of excess estrogen and toxins from the environment in a fatty area devoid of the ability to discharge irritants, spells trouble.

Getting the fat content of your body down to recommended levels will help protect you from breast cancer in many ways. Recent studies show when the fat content of the body is lowered the immune system "revs up." In other words, my immune system would become "mean and lean" and be better at fighting off my breast tumor. Second, studies show that when body fat decreases, estrogen level decreases. Overweight women have much higher levels of estrogen in their body and are more susceptible to breast cancer. I later learned more about which fats are beneficial and aid the immune system and which are toxic or harmful, which I will go into further in Chapter 14.

Below is a chart prepared by Mike Cole at the YMCA according to "The Y's Way to Physical Fitness." Normal body fat content for males and females are 16 and 23 percent, respectively.

Female:	Age Range	Low	High
	12-30	20%	26%
	31-40	21%	27%
	41-50	22%	28%
	51-60	22%	30%
	61+	22%	31%

As this chart indicates, the older we get, the more tissue we lose, the more our body "goes to fat." These figures suggest that the older we get, the harder we have to work at exercising and cutting down the fat content of our diet in order to stay healthy. Fat-to-lean ratio is measured in three ways: electrodes are attached to the feet and water content is measured on a computer; the skin is pulled away and measured with calipers, or the body is immersed in water to measure its bouyancy.

The "Y" will give you a test. This exam is also available

at most other gyms. It can be taken every six months.

A very low fat/lean content is found in women athletes who often get down to seventeen percent or less. A ratio of only eleven to twelve percent however, eliminates so much estrogen that the menstrual period often stops. This happens also in anorexic women. So there is a proportion that is "too low."

One of my friends, Laura, is keeping her fat content down to seventeen percent. She is thin and muscular from her daily work-out with weights, but she is healthy and her periods have not stopped. Since her Mother had breast cancer, she is very careful to eliminate fats in her diet. So far, at forty-eight, her breasts are healthy, even though in her business she is under heavy daily stress. (Postscript: at age forty-nine she did contract breast cancer making this subject even more complex.) The heavy stress she was under and how she carried it within her upper torso may, with her genetic propensity, have contributed to the disease. She had a "C posture"—rounded shoulders, hunched back, along with a deficient diet at the time. This is all, of course, speculation. She had a light case of intraductal carcinoma and sailed through with minimal surgery, keeping her breast and her health.

This morning on TV, an Italian author spoke about her war novel and her breast cancer. As she movingly told the interviewer about her anxiety concerning war, she crossed her arms in front of her chest and rounded her back cradling her tensions within, looking tormented. At the same time, she chain smoked. Were her own physical and mental habits detrimental to the health of this talented lady?

We cannot discount high body fat content. Since the Japanese switched their diet to a more American-European one (fried chicken, ice cream, French pastries—instead of fish, rice, soybeans, and sea-vegetables), their breast cancer rate has soared fifty-eight percent!

Men's body fat is much lower, ranging from twelve to twenty-one percent for a normal, healthy male. Men do get breast cancer but it accounts for only one percent. In males, although it is extremely rare, breast cancer is far more deadly. One out of every twenty-five hundred men will experience the disease.

Under-eating also seems to "rev up" the immune system. Fasting used to be commonly prescribed to heal colds and other diseases.

As well as being extremely low in fats (we only need two-to-five tablespoons of fat a day, whereas the average American diet can go up to as high as forty percent) an increase in fiber has been found to be extremely beneficial. High intake of fiber helps the body eliminate estrogen and lowers breast cancer rate in populations where it is a large part of the diet. Fiber also helps reduce the amount of fat absorbed by the body as it aids in elimination.

The picture I was beginning to get from my readings was the necessity of changing a soft, gooey, "melt-in-your-mouth" sweet, fatty, processed, tenderized, and predigested greasy diet to a minimal coarser, fresher, leaner, and "less affluent" way of eating. I had to eat foods that I had to chew! I had not only to vigorously exercise, I had to vigorously eat!

The soft, cozy way of American life, of licking the plate clean, had to be replaced by a "pioneer spirit"—drier, crunchier diet sans rich sauces, creamy gravies, well-marbled steak, ice cream, and other fats.

My diet at the time was not all that bad. I had already eliminated most but not all dairy products. However, I ate too much meat. I loved meat and ate it almost every day.

Although the bleak picture forming in my mind of a diet of beans and brown rice (not, at that time, my favorite dishes) accompanied by large salads (which I love) was not all that appealing, I have come to slowly readust my tastes. I now love the diet. This takes time. If you are not in a danger zone with a lump already in your breast or elsewhere in your body, I would suggest taking several months to slowly change your concept of eating. We were all mostly raised on the American diet, a diet that even the local American market admits causes several major diseases. (Lucky Market's "Smart Eating" pamphlet is an example of one such confession.) If you aren't Japanese, take time to readust. But readusting may be the best plan if you want to keep your breasts and your health.

Going off caffeine may cause withdrawal symptoms. This might happen also if you eat a lot of sugar. Switching to abundant amounts of raw fruits and vegetables may cause diarrhea at first if you are used to a soft, processed foods diet. So unless you have an emergency situation, go slow.

This diet, then is loaded with fresh fruits and vegetables, eaten raw or lightly cooked, some fish, and lots of grains. No processed foods including canned, frozen, salted, smoked, cured, or pre-made are included if possible. An exception can be made once-in-a-while for canned products such as beans and tuna fish. Refined white flour, sugar, or bakery products made with these are eliminated. Only whole grain/low fat products are acceptable. Few if any dairy products are included for the daily diet. Exceptions are made when entertaining or going out.

Sounds tough? At first it was. Now it seems natural. I no longer hanker after greasy, rich foods and don't miss the meat. Low fat desserts are included if they are made without lots of hydrogenated fats or dairy products. Honey, maple syrup, molasses, or fruit juice are good, natural sweeteners.

I did not try herbs or any special teas or preparations. However, I would like to mention a few: aloe-vera juice, chapparal, sharks cartilage, shitake mushrooms, green tea, and Essiac tea, made from an old Indian recipe for a cancer remedy, are all being experimented with and used by the alternative community. I did add flax seed oil to my diet.

The preparation of food is easier with the following appliances: juicer, blender, wok, cake-rack, chinese-knife (cleaver), and rice cooker.

Breakfast and lunch were fairly simple. It was dinner that proved to be the challenge. The time in which you eat dinner is important. Eating late (after eight p.m. or nine p.m.) when the body is already shutting down for the day means much of what you eat will be converted to fat. Try to eat earlier: at six p.m. or seven p.m.

Here are some typical menus with preparation suggestions when needed. Though this diet was designed for prevention and healing and not as a gourmet adventure, as you go along and experiment, you can find ways to make this food innovative and delicious.

BREAKFASTS:

Fresh squeezed orange juice and vitamin supplements. Sliced fresh fruit topped with a sprinkling of good quality granola without preservatives. I enjoy ones that include whole grains, nuts, and seeds. This is good without milk. Or soy milk or nut milk is a good substitute. Herb tea.

Or: Orange juice, cooked old-fashioned oatmeal with currants or fresh fruit. Herb tea.

Or: Half a grapefruit, wedge of canteloupe or watermelon

(eating some of the seeds), whole grain bread, nut bread, or bran muffin. Herb tea.

Or: Tangerine juice, French toast made with whole grain bread, soaked in two eggs and soy milk or water, cooked in a small amount of butter or safflower oil. Serve with pure maple syrup or fresh fruit. Chinese green tea.

Other breakfast suggestions: whole grain waffles, "instant" breakfast of tofu in a blender with bananas, peaches, cinnamon, nutmeg, and enough apple juice to liquify, rice or barley pudding made with soy milk and served with fresh fruit sweetened with a bit of honey, or whole grain bagels and fruits.

LUNCH:

Packing a lunch everyday to the studio, I made sandwiches out of whole grain bread filled with a combination of vegetables such as avocado and sprouts. (Avocado did not affect the fat content of my body or its ability to throw off the tumors contrary to the advice given in the book, *Doctor's Anti-Cancer Diet.*) Avocado also kept my skin adequately oiled. I have since met a skin-care specialist, Nance Mitchell, who complained that people on the Pritikin diet who ate no fats had dried-out skin. After a good look at my face, she asked me point blank if I ate avocados.

Other good fillings include hummus (mashed garbanzo beans) and zucchini or cabbage. Tuna fish is an old stand-by but I get it packed in water and skipped the mayo. I load the sandwich with lettuce and perhaps a bit of red onion. Three or four fresh fruits are packed along with the sandwich such as apples (non-shiny), peaches, mangos, or persimmons—whatever is in season. A big bottle of spring water joins this lunch and me at the studio all day. Or I'll bring last night's leftover dinner of grains and vegetables in a container, ending the meal with several raw fruits.

Lunch at home or at a restaurant is a big garden salad or steamed vegetable plate. Bean and vegetable tacos are also a treat.

DINNER:

This was the toughest to figure out. I was used to planning the meal around meat. The first consideration was always what kind of meat which indicated what side dishes would be appropriate. Now I had to change my way of thinking. Grains, the "side-dish" now became the main dish. As far as protein, Americans believe we need lots of it —leading to extreme overdose. Grains contain protein that is actually purer and easier to digest. We are all brain-washed by the meat and dairy industries that we need lots of saturated fat type protein. We don't!

Two days a week I could plan the meal around fish. Here is how I prepare it. Take a Chinese wok and fill it part way with water and put in a cake rack. The water should not reach the rack. Let the water come to a simmer while the fish and vegetables are being prepared for steaming. Wash off the fish and put lots of fresh chopped garlic and ginger-root and/or cilantro or dill on top of it. Set it on the rack along with vegetables such as broccoli, green beans, squash, corn on the cob, zucchini, or a wedge of cabbage. Choose two or three vegetables. Grind some black pepper and squeeze some fresh lemon all over. Cover with wok top and let steam for five to ten minutes. Dinner is served.

If corn on the cob is not in season, a half hour before cooking the fish put some rice in the rice cooker. Or try millet, couscous, bulgur, or barley. As an alternative, boil some water in a pot and add some Japanese buckwheat noodles, or whole grain pasta. This is "fast-food" at its best. Steaming brings out the flavor of very fresh fish so it doesn't need a sauce. Steamed vegetables, besides being more nutritious than boiled, taste better. There are lots of terrific kinds of fish that do very well steamed: trout, salmon, sword-fish, mahi-mahi, halibut, catfish, cod, sole, or red-snapper to name a few. If you like hot food, slice a thumbnail size red-pepper and top with hot spice before steaming. Experiment with different herbs such as rosemary or basil. Soy sauce is also a good flavor enhancer. Experiment with whole grains from around the world.

Pasta is usually a favorite with everybody. It can be bought fresh or dried at the market. It's also fun to make it yourself. Look for semolina flour or whole-grain pasta rather than the white-flour product which is non-nutritious. For a sauce, cook down some fresh tomatoes such as Italian plum, in some olive oil into which a couple of garlic cloves have been added. Season with oregano, basil, parsley, onions, or whatever you like. Or make my favorite—a pesto sauce. Get two or three bunches of fresh basil and put them into a blender with a couple of handfuls of pine nuts, some olive oil and two cloves of garlic, some parsley, and ground black pepper. Grind to a paste. Toss with freshly cooked pasta in a hot wok. This is a really delicious dinner. Serve with a big tossed salad.

A terrific lasagna can be made with vegetables such as spinach and zucchini layered with canned tomato sauce and baked in the oven. I don't miss the cheese at all.

Even pizza can be made with a whole wheat or corn flour crust and embellished with different toppings. Try experimenting with various vegetables and mushrooms and canned tomato sauce. Tofu can be crumbled and put on an oiled baking sheet and browned in the oven for half-an-hour to substitute for ground beef.

Experiment with different squashes or broiled eggplant. Skip the cheese. You don't need it.

One thing I really love making is polenta. Find some coarse Italian cornmeal especially for polenta in a specialty market. Bring three cups of water to boiling in a saucepan. Combine one cup of polenta with two cups of water and gradually wisk this corn-meal mixture into the boiling water.

Reduce heat to low and stir while cooking it for thirty minutes. It will become very thick. Season with salt and pepper. Pour into an oiled nine inch glass pie plate and refrigerate until firm.

Polenta is great served with a sauce of stir-fried wilted greens cooked in garlic, or a tomato sauce. It can also be toasted in a little olive oil to warm it again before serving.

Before going to bed one night, soak some beans in water. Dried beans taste better than canned. Beans make great stews, soups, and even salads. The next day when you are ready to cook the beans, throw out the water. Add new water and cook for about one-and-a-quarter hours. Season with chiles, chili powder, cilantro, tomatoes, garlic, onions, bell pepper, and/or squash.

This bean stew can be served with rice and a mixed green salad. I like a simple dressing made out of a good grade olive oil, flax seed oil, balsamic vinegar (it is expensive—but a little goes a long way), a little lemon juice and some raw garlic pressed through a garlic press. I don't like bottled dressings which always taste flat to me. Fresh garlic is a known tumor-fighter.

If you don't have time to soak and cook beans you can resort to canned. Chickpeas and lentils are good canned. These beans also contain Laetrile. Throw chickpeas into salads or make a bean stew or soup with them. Lentils and black beans, as well as vegetarian baked beans, make great fillers for tacos. Use corn or whole-wheat tortillas rather than flour, and fill with beans, lettuce, tomatoes, cilantro, guacamole (fresh avocado, mashed and mixed with green onions and smashed garlic, chopped tomato, and lemon or lime juice). Stir-fried fish cut into bite-size pieces is also a great addition to these tacos. Instead of sour cream, throw some tofu in a blender with lemon juice. It even tastes a bit like sour cream! You won't miss the cheese as these are so good.

I like to experiment with different grains. Barley is not only my favorite, but it is without rival for cancer healing and prevention. Barley can be cooked in a rice cooker. Or simmer one cup of barley in three cups of water for one-and-a-quarter hours. Top with stir-fried vegetables cooked in olive oil that has been seasoned with fresh garlic. (Heat the wok, then put in a couple tablespoons of oil, heat that, then throw in the garlic. The vegetables can then be added. Barley makes great soups—and puddings, too. It is also included in some cooked cereals such as Kashi. It is loaded with Laetrile. Barley is perhaps, the oldest grain, cultivated in China two thousand years ago. Eating this grain is very comforting. It gives a wonderful, "full" feeling.

Rice can be made into a main dish rissoto, or stir-fried with vegetables. Brown and wild rice taste better than the more refined white rice. Rice can also be made into soups or puddings.

A main dish of scalloped potatoes can be easily made using a tofu and lemon ''cream'' sauce. Slice new potatoes with skin on. Stir-fry in the wok and then cover and steam until tender. Add the sauce (tofu and lemon combined in a blender) and toss. Season with ground black pepper.

Try to find the best produce and splurge. It's the best health insurance. Buy stone-ground flour in small bags and keep refrigerated. Use olive oil for cooking. Olive oil, nut oil, or flax seed oil are good for dressings. Bypass heavier saturated fats such as butter, lard, bacon fat, and hydrogenated shortenings such as Crisco. Even pie crust can be made with oil. Margarine is an over-processed plasticized fat devoid of nutritional value that should be avoided.

I'm giving you some ideas to get started, if you haven't considered a vegetarian diet before. It's my belief that if every women went on this diet beginning early in life, we would see a very drastic cut in the current spiraling of breast cancer statistics.

If you are currently fighting breast cancer or breast lumps or if you want to help prevent recurrence, this diet will really help. As we say in Buddhism, this diet is based on ''actual proof.'' It helped me slough off my breast and uterine tumors and continued to help me improve my health. It's also a great diet for losing weight or in maintaining weight. Eliminating most fat, you will find you don't gain weight as easily. The "yo-yo" effect of always gaining and losing the same pounds is eliminated.

You don't even have to cut out dessert. I eat lots of dates which are loaded with Vitamin A. Other fruits, especially red, yellow, or orange, can be eaten fresh or baked into goods made with whole grain flour. If you don't want to bake, there are now organic fat-free cookies on the market.

Here are some cookbooks to get you started:

One of the best, because it does not use dairy products, is *Friendly Foods* by Brother Ron Pickarski, O.F.M. This is a gourmet vegetarian cuisine compilation published by Ten Speed Press, Berkeley, California. I met the author at a health-food convention in Anaheim, California and tasted one of his desserts which was outstanding.

Natural Healing Cookbook by Mark Bricklin and Sharon Classens, 1981, Rodale Press, Emmarus, Penn. has a section on breast lumps and a study showing why the elimination of caffeine (coffee, tea—not herb or Chinese Green Tea—chocolate, and colas) is important. It has a terrific recipe for Carrot-Apricot soup.

Great Tasting Health Foods by Robert Rodale published by "Prevention Magazine" is a good resource. The *Tassajara Recipe Book* by Edward Espe Brown Boston, Shambhala, 1985, has tips on how to make tofu taste good by marinating it. It also has a good garbanzo stew. However, the recipes use dairy products, so it needs to be experimented with.

Diet for a Small Planet by Frances Moor Lappe, is a classic work—a vegetarian bible—with instructions on food combining and a chapter on the "protein myth." Again, it uses some dairy products. Soy products can be substituted most of the time. Vegetarians have less osteoporosis. Digesting dairy products robs calcium from the bones contrary to what the dairy industry would have us believe. Chinese women eat no dairy products. Osteoporosis is virtually unknown in that country.

Mollie Katzen writes two vegetarian cookbooks. *The Moosewood Cookbook* and *The Enchanted Broccoli Forest*, Ten Speed Press, Berkeley, California, have good sections on grains and vegetables. Again, eliminate dairy products. Katzen has updated her books in a new edition that incorporates less fat in her recipes.

Two books on using Tofu have been quite useful. *Tofu Magic* by Julia Weinberg, Westwood, CA., Cookwrite Publishing, 1988, has everything from Broccoli Soup to Pizza and Honey-Lemon Un-cheese cake. Some dairy products are used which can be eliminated.

Nasoya foods puts out *Tofu Cookbook* which has a good ratatouille recipe. Michio Kushi of the East West Foundation explains the macrobiotic diet in the *Macrobiotic Approach to Cancer*, Wayne, New Jersey, Avery Publishing Co., which shows how to discover your own cooking style while using foods that prevent and eliminate cancer. From the same publishing company comes Marcea Weber's *Naturally Sweet Desserts* which has everything from apple pie to vanilla ice cream made without sugar or dairy products. Artificial ingredients found in commercial ice cream are discussed such as Amylacetate—used for banana flavoring and also as a paint solvent. In the foreword there is a story of how a patient got rid of PMS (pre-menstrual syndrome, enlarged breasts, and fluid retention) when she eliminated sugar, caffeine, and all dairy products from her diet.

There are many other good vegetarian cookbooks and health-food cookbooks. I have listed a few to get you started. I've also found Chinese cookbooks, in general, very helpful. India has a marvelous vegetarian cuisine to explore.

I also subscribe to "Food and Wine" magazine. A good article on bean cookery was featured in the March 1991 issue. In this issue, I also read about how lowering dietary fats "revs" up the immune system. This news was in their "Healthy Eating" section by Jeanine Barone in their timely, for me, February 1991 issue. I was in the midst of my battle at that time. Paradoxically, to sell the magazine, the cover features steak and french fries!

Needless to say, this isn't a health-food magazine, but they do have a department that regularly covers low calorie cooking. Their "Healthy Eating" news seems to always have interesting tips and facts.

When eating out, I pick Chinese, Indian, Thai, or Japanese restaurants. Some contemporary American restaurants now serve "nouvelle cuisine" which is often low fat.

Mexican restaurants often cook with lard, but they may have things you can order such as their soup with warm tortillas. Mexicans also have less breast cancer with their high-fiber diet that features beans and rice and corn tortillas.

Its a good idea to avoid "fast-food" drive-ins, or greasy-spoons, and steak houses (when in doubt, order fish and/or a salad).

To summarize, the MOTEP diet emphasizes whole grains, fruits and vegetables eaten raw or lightly cooked. Fish, nuts and seeds, legumes, and tofu are included. (Shell fish is alright, although you should watch out for shrimp—some people get shingles from its high uretic acid content. Others, like me, have inherited gout and can have an attack from eating too much shrimp).

This diet eliminates all meat, dairy products, refined white flour and sugar, and caffeine, and most alcohol—except an occasional glass of wine. It emphasizes foods rich in Vitamin A, B17, C, E, and Selenium. This diet not only helps prevent and eliminate breast lumps, helps heal cancer, but also will change your appearance rather drastically to a beautiful new you!

Don't be rigid or pedantic about this diet. Find out what

works for you. If you are invited to a party where the hostess proudly serves her Chinese Chicken Salad, go ahead and eat it. Enjoying life is part of the MOTEP program. You can always go back to your special diet the next day. To your health.

Bon Appetite!!

Don't Eat Plastic **9**

When Meryl Streep led an organization called "Mothers and Others," formed to protest pesticide used on our fruits and vegetables, she got action. Mainly targeting Daminozide, sold under the name of Alar, a chemical used on apples to promote their growth, her campaign aimed at stopping the effects on children who were found to develop cancer from ingesting this toxin.

I joined her movement. For ten years prior to her campaign, I had been on my apple bandwagon. I had been trying to alert everyone I could about the fact that often plastic was now being used to "protect, preserve, and beautify" apples instead of the traditional wax which had become economically unfeasible to use.

Compared to my feeble efforts (although I now see fewer sprayed apples in the markets where I shop and complain about groceries), Meryl was strikingly successful. It seemed in short order that Alar was totally banned. (1989)

In Los Angeles the school system even took up the cause and banned apples for a few days. We are very loyal to our movie stars since this is a "Hollywood" town. A few days later, however, the School Board questioned this decision getting confused and deciding banning apples would be like prohibiting Mothers. They then reinstated them.

When "Mothers and Others" began its campaign I signed up, just another of the millions against pesticide use never knowing someday I would meet Meryl. But one evening I received this tremendous opportunity.

Being an artist has somehow made me interesting to movie stars, who after all, are artists themselves. Meryl was at a crowded, lively opening at an Art Gallery in Santa Monica. As I rounded the corner I saw a glimpse of her memorable face. She was dressed simply and wore no make-up. In a late stage of pregnancy with her fourth child, her quiet beauty and classic features still took my breath away as it never fails to do when I see her on the screen.

She was surrounded by her husband and a denizen of collectors and gallery people. I thought I had not a chance to meet her. Fortunately, one of this elite crowd recognized me. In fact, she hugged me.

Meryl smiled and looked my way. Sensing this was my chance, I grabbed her hand.

"Oh, Meryl, I just want to tell you that you are my most favorite, in the whole world, actress. When you are on the screen there is a luminous quality about you: you light up the screen as no other actor or actress can do!"

She took all this outpouring with the quiet dignity she always possesses. Unruffled, though obviously pleased, she began to empathize with me on the subject of how hard it was for an artist to be at their own opening!

When she spoke, the warmth and electricity radiated from her inner being and her plain, pale face filled with color and beauty. We conversed a bit more. A friendship was begun. But soon there were other people for her to see. I had to leave without getting in a good apple discussion.

She *was* interested in knowing about the spray coating used on apples and other fruits and vegetables, or as one grocer termed it, "food grade shellac" when I talked to her at another party. Perhaps she would turn her star power on helping us to eliminate this carcinogenic processing of apples and other fruits and vegetables. She also narrated a television special about Rachel Carson's book, *Silent Spring,* an early warning about the dangers of DDT.

While waiting for Meryl to come center stage on this issue, we as consumers can use our collective buying power to vote by "just saying NO" to super-glossy apples, cucumbers, zucchini, strawberries, oranges, bell-peppers, squash, cherries, and any other glossy fruits and vegetables.

These could be coated with plastic that cannot be scratched or washed off. Peeling is not an altogether safe alternative either, since skin is semi-permeable and lets plastic through.

As we are learning with breast implants, the plastic does not aimlessly float around in the body as I originally imagined. It is attacked and broken down to its component parts, one which is the solvent toluene, stronger than turpentine which causes cancer of the liver. Who knows if this irritant can also work its way up the breast and cause enough damage to a gene to destroy its ability to replicate breast tissue and mutate it to the point that it can only be able to reproduce itself?

At a recent lecture at UCLA, Dr. Susan Love revealed she is now finding PCB's (plastic particles) in the breasts of some of her cancer patients during surgery.

And where are you on this issue, David Kessler? He is our new FDA chief who is beginning to get a reputation as being tough. Following a mandate that an orange juice distributor take the "fresh" labeling off its container after finding they actually stored the juice in a warehouse for two weeks, he surprised me (after this token effort) by going after breast implants—giving me hope for the future.

The issue of chemicalized and plasticized foods which in all probability contribute to the one million cancer cases each year, half of which lead to death, seems of momentous importance. Working to eliminate carcinogenic substances from our food supply would certainly help to stop this alarming epidemic. According to Bill Moyer, author of *Healing and the Mind,* the EPA has only cracked down on nineteen of the over six-hundred carcinogenic chemicals used by farmers in growing our food!

The use of hormones to fatten beef and chicken and increase milk production in dairy cows is also an issue of momentous importance. Cows treated with a new experimental growth hormone, "Recombinant Bovine Growth Hormone" (sounds like DES all over again) have been found to come down with mastitis, an inflammation of the udder. These cows are then treated with antibiotics to "cure" this hormone-caused disease. These hormones and antibiotics are then passed along to the consumer in meat and milk. If a hormone will irritate and inflame a cow's breast, think of the possibilities for women who drink this milk!

There is actually a law which has been on the books for fifty years that companies have to label what they spray on fruit and vegetables. However, this information has only to be written on the crate and not passed on to the consumer. The shopper is attracted to these items precisely because of their glamorous appearance. These "designer" items should be labeled with a skull and cross-bones. The modern grocery store has become no longer a "safe-way" but rather a purveyor of many varieties of various poisons and carcinogenic substances disguised in and around what used to be food.

How did we get to this sorry state where commercial interests in selling chemicals usurped our interest in nutrition and health? How has the cancer rate jumped from one out of six people in the forties to become one out of three people in the nineties with a prognosis for the future of one out of two or half of us becoming ill with cancer by the year two thousand?

Some light on this subject was shed for me at the Nineteenth Annual Cancer Convention in Pasadena, California. I learned that you can actually buy apricot pits in a health food store so you don't have to use a hammer to obtain Laetrile in this country. They even had for sale, a recipe book on how to use them. *(The Little Cyanide Cookbook—Delicious Recipes Rich in Vitamin B17)* by June de Spain, American Media 1976). When I went to the health food store to buy apricot kernels, I learned that supplements made from this nutrient were banned by the FDA some years ago. They no longer can carry the anti-cancer substance in pill form. The clerk told me this was to aid in sale of chemotherapy drugs!

On August 31, 1991, Mark Anderson, author of *Empty Harvest* spoke at the convention on modern food production. Synthetic fertilizers, he noted, were first invented by a German named Justus von Liebig. These fertilizers do not give life to the soil as manure and composting do but create an oil-based agriculture that causes plants to grow despite bad, lifeless soil. This soil merely holds the plant in a vertical position without giving them the vitamins and minerals they need to become healthy. These puny, diseased plants have lost their natural immunity to insects and thus are attacked. Mother nature wants to get rid of them! More chemicals are then used as pesticides to kill off the insects and molds. These weak diseased plants that somehow, through modern chemistry, still resemble normal, healthy fruits and vegetables, are further beautified with plastic to make them shiny and pretty. In the final stage, they are trucked to the grocery store for the unwary consumer, namely us.

What's in a name? Justus von Liebig. He started it. We finish it by buying a big, red, shiny apple and go home to eat it only to find a tasteless, toxic product that will not nourish our cells, but will, in fact, poison us. What the chemical companies and farm products producers and grocers have done is banded together to LIE BIG.

(Ironically, Liebig in German means "loving.")

In order to produce healthy cells in our body, we need oxygen from the air (a now rare commodity), water which is clean and pure (practically extinct), and enzymes, vitamins and minerals from fresh, unprocessed, unrefined, and unpoisoned food.

This seems to be a tall order in today's commercially-oriented society bent on preserving profits. The goal is sales:

selling a lot of chemicals and petroleum products. As a result, people's health breaks down. They get cancer. This leads to more sales of surgery, cutting up their bodies, along with sales of more toxic chemicals and radiation—more and more poisons trying to rectify the illnesses they got from poisoning in the first place! Using poisons to combat poisoning is some sort of absurd logic only the medical profession and the drug companies could understand!

Is it surprising that this "treatment" only makes people sicker and compounds their pain and suffering?

The Hunza people who eat apricot pits also fertilize their own soil. They allow no imported food. They don't get cancer and are some of the longest-lived people in the world.

Headline in the "Los Angeles Times" the other day, Friday, September 6, 1991: "Partial Ban on Lethal Pesticide Parathion O.K.'d." This means by the end of the year the Environmental Protection Agency will make sure that only fifty percent of the three million to six million pounds of parathion sprayed on about ninety U.S. crops each year be used. Under the voluntary agreement, parathion cannot be used after December 31, 1991 on such crops as apples, almonds, oats, peaches, and peanuts though it will take eighteen months to force an end to the remaining nine uses: alfalfa, barley, canola, corn, cotton, sorghum, soybeans, sunflower, and wheat. These account for an estimated forty to fifty percent of all parathion use in this country.

At the top of the article some background is given for this chemical. "Developed in Germany in World War II, parathion is a chemical cousin of deadly agents used by the Nazis during the Holocaust. Because of its low cost, it became a widely used pesticide for ninety different crops even though it was considered the most dangerous because of the poisoning of farm workers. In cases of a small mistake, the worker might get a lethal exposure.

We now have moved past discrimination. Instead of poisoning only Jews, we now include Catholics, Protestants, Christians, Buddhists, and everyone else in America regardless of race or creed who buys and eats these fruits, vegetables, nuts, and beans. Using his ideas and products, we've surpassed Hitler in our abilities of extermination! The cancer rate climbs steadily continuing to obliterate our precious good health and life itself.

In Los Angeles, we have regularly had to submit to whole sections of the city being sprayed with Malathion in order to combat the Mediterranean Fruit Fly that supposedly would destroy our fruit crop. Helicopters buzz menacingly over our heads at night spraying this poison over everybody (people!) with only the warning that we should cover our cars. Malathion curdles paint enamel. We are also told to bring in our outdoor fish aquariums as the spray kills fish! This lethal spraying of whole populations, not just fruit, was fought bitterly by citizens, many who got ill. The fight was spearheaded by my friend, Councilman Joel Wachs, who is also an avid art collector.

When I found an article in a book describing Malathion as a derivative of Nazi poisons originally designed to obliterate human beings, I referred it to Joel. Still his efforts did not stop the spraying until much later. Crickets and many birds were killed off. Far worse, it may have planted the seeds of many cancer cases down the line. The fact is, cancer sometimes takes twenty years or more to gestate.

Ralph Moss, whom I finally got to briefly meet, spoke at the cancer convention. He came up with this startling bit of information: THERE ARE NOW FIVE HUNDRED MILLION POUNDS OF SYNTHETIC CHEMICALS IN OUR ENVIRONMENT.

These chemicals are in our food, our air, our oceans, and our drinking water!

Although basically our bodies have not changed since the Pleistocene age, we are now in the Plastic age. Physically, we were not designed to ingest petroleum-based plastics, breathe petroleum products, or have plastics inserted into our bodies!

We are becoming consciously aware consumers. The trend is to want ORGANIC fruits and vegetables as well as grains that are grown without the use of chemical fertilizers, pesticides, fungicides, and other chemical sprays. We need tougher laws to discourage synthetic chemicals being used in food production.

We know in order to avoid breast cancer, we must eat at least five servings of vegetables and fruits a day—up to fifty percent of our diet. How can we make sure what we are buying and eating is safe, nutritional, and non-toxic?

One way to start is to hold that vegetable or fruit you are thinking of putting in our grocery cart up to the light. See if it sparkles with a high gloss that used to be reserved for your candy-apple red Ford you bought as a teenager. Take a fingernail to that glossy surface and see if you can scratch through it. If you can't, the possibility of plastic being used is very high. Take it over to the manager or the produce fellow and ask if this sort of coating can be washed off. If he assures you it can, let him water it down and show you. If it doesn't wash and if his "perfectly harmless" story doesn't wash either, complain vociferously and refuse to buy it. This is the only way we can begin to affect change. **We, the consumers, must use our voices and our wallets to stop practices of poisoning currently used by the food industry.**

Early detection of breast cancer with its emphasis on mammograms should be changed to "early prevention" beginning with the food we eat. We should be thinking about ways to stop trouble before it starts rather than how to detect it when it already may be too late.

Through a group called the "Edge" which supplied me with my group therapy, I met Dr. Earl Mindell who kindly sent me his book, *Unsafe at Any Meal*. This book is a sort of gruesome dictionary of three thousand additives and plastic materials the government permits manufacturers to add or use as ingredients while still maintaining that the product is "food" and safe to eat. He also chronicles the adverse reactions, diseases, and allergies these additives can cause. For instance BHA and BHT which stand for Butylated hydroxyanisole and Butylated hydroxytoluene (remember toluene, that toxic thinner we discussed earlier?) can lead to the possible adverse effects of elevated cholesterol levels, allergic reactions, liver damage, infertility, sterility, behavior problems, loss of Vitamin D, weakened immune system, and increased susceptibility to cancer-causing substances.

A quick grocery store tour will reveal these poisons. For instance, "BHT is added to the packaging material to preserve freshness" is written on the box of a popular brand of cereal, Post, with a "back to nature" photo on the front.

In other words, we are feeding a noxious plastics-thinner I refuse to use in the studio to thin paints, as a morning breakfast food to our children!

A popular whipped topping revealed the following plastic additives: sodium casinate, polysorbate sixty, monosterearate, artificial flavors, as well as other "ingredients." Even the natural components of this whipped topping, hydrogenated coconut and palm kernel oils (high in fats) and white sugar turn this topping into a health-threatening dessert enhancement.

How are these poisons related to cancer? Linus Pauling, twice a Nobel Prize winner, relates in his book, *Cancer and Vitamin C* which he wrote with Ewan Cameron, "Man is under a constant bombardment from a hail of potentially lethal carcinogens. These are a whole variety of physical and chemical agents that share one common property—the ability to interact with and to damage the genetic material of living cells. Such damage may, on a million-to-one chance, damage and rearrange the genetic material in such a way that the offspring of the transformed cell can survive and also acquire malignant characteristics (rather than being completely killed off by the carcinogen)." (p. 184).

Another explanation came at the cancer convention where I met Charlotte Gerson whose father, Max Gerson, M.D., treated terminally ill cancer patients given up by the medical establishment after their treatments failed and they were sent home to die. She sold me her father's book, *A Cancer Therapy—Results of Fifty Cases and the Cure of Advanced Cancer by Diet Therapy.*

Dr. Gerson was adamantly against symptomatic treatment which he thought was harmful (cutting a lump out of a breast, cutting off a breast). He believed that cancer is a disease of the entire metabolism concentrated essentially in the liver which cannot filter through accumulated poisons ingested and inhaled into the system when, over a period of time, their cumulative effect is overwhelming. As the body becomes more poisoned it becomes more reduced in its defense and healing power. (p. 7).

Cancer, then, in Gerson's view, is a chronic, degenerative disease affecting all essential organs in which the body is so poisoned it cannot produce mature cells but instead produces cells in the embryonic state which cannot function except to reproduce themselves.

Rather than treat a disease, Max Gerson approached cancer patients as sick human beings. He treated the person.

He writes, "It should always be borne in mind that cancer is a degenerative disease. The regeneration is only possible through the metabolism. Its restoration is hard work, but is essential and the last refuge for these advanced cases." (p. 112).

Gerson's treatment consisted chiefly of freshly squeezed juices given every hour and coffee enemas to clean out the body. Slowly, a mostly raw fruit and vegetable diet was introduced and a vegetable soup from a recipe by Hippocrates! It should be noted that some of his patients came in on stretchers and could not eat at all.

His book documents fifty cases of cured cancer—all these cases were rejected by the medical establishment after treatment failures.

Of interest here is case number thirty-three, Mrs. M. E., age sixty-two, a widow with one child, who had an ulceration of the right breast below the nipple. The right nipple was somewhat retracted and indurated. Below the lateral areola edge was a firm, palpable mass. X-rays of the lung were negative.

Condition when first seen already showed an open ulcer formation and large infiltrating mass. Patient had refused an operation.

After four weeks of detox treatment, the infiltration was barely palpable and the ulcer was covered with a fine crust. The patient was healing. Nipple, however, was still retracted. The next month, no infiltration was felt and the ulcer was closed. Nipple slightly retracted. Nine months later the nipple was partially everted, no other changes.

The patient had no recurrence and seven years later was driving a car and doing housework. The patient had no other treatment before Gerson saw her or after. (p. 349).

As I write this chapter, my friend Kimberly is going into the hospital for the Medical Establishment's idea of a "last-ditch" treatment, an autologous bone marrow transplant. Today, bone marrow will be taken out of her pelvis. Next week she will undergo five to seven days of extraordinarily high-dose heavy-duty toxic chemotherapy to "kill" the cancer cells after which her bone marrow will be reinserted.

She will be in the hospital a total of six weeks which is what is required to recuperate from such an exposure to highly toxic chemicals. Both Dr. David Clark and I opposed this form of treatment when she suggested she might submit herself to it. David said that bone marrow transplants were usually reserved for leukemia patients and never done on any patient over thirty-five. Kimberly is now thirty-seven.

When I asked her husband, Gerry, for statistics on this procedure, he said this was an "experimental" treatment and the only statistics he knew were that fifteen percent of the patients used to die from the treatment. Now that they've improved it, only three percent die from it! (According to the UCLA Breast Center five to twenty percent of bone marrow patients die from bone marrow transplants.)

He could only tell me that a rare case was put into remission from this treatment. "But," he said, "it's all they know."

The startlingly horrifying fact that came out at the cancer convention is that there are no double-blind studies done on chemotherapy.

Linus Pauling questions the use of chemotherapy because it kills off all fast-growing cells such as bone marrow cells. Whenever the immune system is destroyed there is an *increased* risk of getting cancer.

One rationalization I have read from various doctors for

using chemotherapy is that it keeps patients oriented toward the medical and away from "quacks and charletans!"

In two weeks, I will be able to visit her at the Cancer Center at which time I will experience for myself, cancer first-hand as treated by the Orthodox methods in a hospital setting. Already I am praying for her and bracing myself to see some very, very sick debilitated people, one of whom is my long-time friend whom I love. Will I feel they are murdering her? Will I scream out, "Stop this massacre! This is wrong! She doesn't need anymore poison!" Will they have to escort me bodily out in a straight-jacket as I flail out wildly at the doctors?

(For a vivid description of Chemotherapy treatment, see the film "Dying Young" with Julia Roberts).

As for me, when Dr. Furr found a stone-like lump in my breast, I chose the detoxification route. Not having yet read Dr. Gerson's book, I was yet familiar with juices and limiting my diet to raw and steamed vegetables, fruits, grains, and fish. I shop for them at the highest quality market, read labels, and buy organic foods whenever possible. I eliminated all meat and chicken because of their high fat content, hormones, and antibiotics and because over-dosing on protein is also linked to cancer.

According to Dr. Max Gerson, the purpose of detoxification is to allow the body to produce an inflammatory reaction which then kills the cancer cells. A normal, healthy, non-toxic body can produce this reaction whereas cancer patients could not because their bodies were too toxic. If this is the case, then my own inflammatory breast cancer which happened one month into my self-treatment program was actually a part of my healing process.

Whereas, I thought at the time my inflammed neon-red breast meant that my program wasn't working or that it hadn't kicked in yet, according to Dr. Gerson this meant my program *was* working. This reaction which he calls "flare-ups" is precisely what he aimed at in his detoxification program. The inflammatory reaction heats the body like a fever and dissolves the tumor. Cytokines then swarm around like bees attacking the lump. All these reactions are how the body heals itself of cancer. It is, however, a rather frightening and horrifying experience. You think you are going to die. You get ready to write your last will and testament! (Charlotte Gerson remarked that some cancer patients quit when they see this reaction, becoming alarmed that they are getting worse.)

But three weeks later the tumor dissolved completely and instead of dying, I slowly regained my health. I will continue MOTEP for one-and-a-half years as Dr. Gerson suggests to completely heal. **In fact, I have decided to continue the program for the duration of my life.**

In summary, to avoid the misery and suffering of breast cancer, one thing we must do is to be very alert consumers. Eating chemicalized, plasticized foods full of additives and sprays grown from synthetic oil-based soil devoid of the vitamins and minerals we need will result in the body's breakdown into sickness, disease, and cancer. Read labels, examine produce, complain.

The breast you save may be your own!

Exercise— 10
Dive Into Health

In the movie "L.A. Story," Steve Martin gets into his car to drive two houses down in a row of tract homes!

Contrary to this visual portrayal of a soft, effortless life, Steve Martin, in person has the body of an exercise fanatic with a stomach as taut and flat as a washboard. I met him at (you guessed) an art gallery in Santa Monica where I was currently showing my art. It was a weekday; the gallery was empty, I thought. As I talked to my dealer, Ruth, I glanced over at the corner for a moment. There was Steve Martin walking towards me out of the shadows. I couldn't help staring.

Steve noticed I saw him and headed straight for me. Finally he stopped and began to try to stare me down. I took up the challenge as I consider myself quite strong and able to stare down just about anybody. He was standing quite close and as he is a rather tall, large man with quite a lot of personal power, this was very intimidating. Still, I thought I could handle the situation and stared back. After a while of this staring, I felt an incredible energy focused on my head rather like an electric drill running through it. This became most unbearable and I had to lurch away.

"You're just a _____, I said, not completing my sentence. I turned back to look at Steve who ducked. Maybe he thought I was going to call him by the title of one of his movies ("The Jerk"). I waited. My dealer, Ruth, flinched. I finally finished my sentence. . . ."GREAT ACTOR!"

Steve slowly smiled. He took another step forward and let his right shoulder drop quickly toward me in a pantomime of "let's go!" Steve is actually a very shy man and this whole first meeting was done without his ever saying one word. I did walk with him a while, conversing with words while he used only gestures, facial expressions, and body language; until his silence unnerved and overwhelmed me and I ran off.

It took me two years to get his first sentence out of him at the premiere of his film "L.A. Story" where he said, "I'm very glad you were able to come."

But to get back to exercise, the subject of this chapter, we must first get out of our car and use the legs, arms, and muscles which nature provided us. Her motto seems to be: USE OR LOSE IT. This seems applicable to breast cancer as the highest rate turns up in nuns, unmarried women, married women with no children, and women who had their children later in life. Women who had children early in life, shortly before or after twenty years of age and those that breast-fed their babies have low rates. The usual explanation for this is that pregnancy affords a break in the estrogen cycle which makes the cells proliferate in the milk glands every month until mid-month; when no pregnancy occurs another set of hormones causes the cells to regress. Pregnancy gives this roller-coaster hormonal cycle a rest.

I have another theory to add to this. The breasts may be tired and frustrated! Their job as attractive, modified sweat glands, afterall, is to produce milk each month in readiness to suckle a baby. If we start our cycle at age fourteen and complete it at age fifty without ever having an outlet for this "job," then the breast has prepared its milk-release readiness cycle once a month for thirty-six years or four hundred thirty-two times without having any release or job satisfaction! Talk about weariness and frustration! Toward menopause when this efficient gland sees that after all its preparation for a job it never gets, it now has to retire—well, how would you feel?

Since I decided early in life to devote myself to my art and not have children, a breakdown may have been inevitable. The next best outlet for frustration is exercise. I had a stone-like lump in my breast and a rock in my uterus I had to get rid of myself without resorting to surgery. What I was aiming at was what the Medical Establishment calls "spontaneous regression." This term, to me, is equivalent to "overnight success" in art. That is, after working for twenty years or more, suddenly an important curator or dealer decides to show the work, everyone wants to buy this work the artist has slaved for decades to make, and suddenly, voila, the artist is an "overnight success!"

I'm here to puncture the balloon of "spontaneous regression" and "overnight success."

Both are, in my experience, a lot of "cause and effect" hard, sweaty work!

Everson and Cole, in their book *Spontaneous Regression of Cancer*, document around two hundred cases of cancer which seemingly, magically, suddenly disappeared.[17]

Of interest here is a woman in her sixties who came into the doctor's office with lymphatic cancer, her breast deformed and scarred over in typical carcinoma pattern. She said that when she went through menopause, her breast had "changed shape." But that was seventeen years ago.

We don't know what this lady did to arrest her breast cancer herself and keep it in check for an astounding length of time (or what her body did for her). It would have been interesting to interview her. For now, I can relate to you what I did.

---

[17] Everson, Tilden C. and Cole, Warren H. *Spontaneous Regression of Cancer.* Philadelphia and London. W. B. Saunders. 1966.

In devising my exercise program, then, it had to fulfill several requirements:

1. An aerobic cardio-vascular exercise that would involve the large muscle groups of the chest (pectoral) and upper arms (biceps and triceps) and increase the heart rate and demand for oxygen.

2. One that would pit these muscles against a resistance or workload.

3. One that I could enjoy doing for approximately one hour each day, five to six days a week.

4. One that would decrease the fat-to-lean ratio of my body, that is, eliminate the overly high-fat content. (See chart).

5. One that would allow me to "space out," forget my worries, and use in combination with my visualization exercises.

Swimming satisfies all these requirements for me. If you enjoy swimming, I encourage you to incorporate this wonderful exercise daily into your routine. Swimming is a low risk sport (provided you know how) that uses all muscle groups. It offers a weightless, soothing environment (your body is only ten percent of its weight in water) while providing a constant workload or resistance which the muscles must combat in order to move backward or forward or even to stay in the same place (treading water).

Just for a moment, stand up and put your right hand

above your left breast. Raise your left arm now and go through some strokes you use when you swim: backcrawl, Australian crawl (forward), breast stroke, backstroke, (frog). Feel the muscles you use as you pull your arms up, out, and forcefully down. Sense the tensions loosening that you have perhaps stored in your breast from everyday stress or emotional problems and frustrations. Now do this exercise again this time incorporating a white light coming from your eyes, or "third eye," and visualize this light cleaning and soothing your breast and dissolving forcefully, like a laser-beam, any lumps.

During this exercise you will begin to feel what I did with the added resistance and pleasure of soothing water. Joining a gym or the local "Y" and setting a regular scheduled time of the day, five to six days a week, was one of the most important parts of my self-lumpectomy program. I began slowly as I hadn't been swimming laps for a while. I would swim for forty-five minutes at first. Gradually, I worked up to the mile which took me sixty-five minutes. Finally I was able to accomplish this mile in forty-five minutes.

O.K. I admit I am a swimmer. I was a lifeguard in my teens and also taught swimming. It's my sport. But my "exercise routine" before this new schedule had degenerated into sitting in the steam bath after work.

Go gradually into a vigorous routine if you haven't worked out for a while. Overdoing exercise or pushing yourself too hard before you are ready is very dangerous and can even lead to death. Listen to your body and do as much as you can, then stop. Tomorrow is another day to do a little more. You don't have to start out being Jane Fonda. The benefits of exercise are cumulative and doing a little each day will accomplish more in the long run than sporadic all-out efforts. Slowly, your body will build resistance to disease as it gets stronger. If you already have a lump, or cancer, be patient. Exercise will give your body a valuable tool it needs to re-build healthy cells and destroy malignant ones. THIS TAKES TIME. Be assured that your body is working to regain its health. The more you work, the more ammunition you are giving it to self-heal.

You may not like to swim. It's important to do exercise that you enjoy. Other sports that might qualify are archery, rowing (or a rowing machine), basketball, weights, and nautilus machines. The seated chest press, behind-the-neck pull, double-shoulder, multi-biceps, multi-triceps, military press, and free weights are all breast health promoters. These machines involve the arms and pectoral muscles beneath the breasts to push, lift, expand, and contract. You are building strength, endurance, resistance to erosion by cancerous cells, and healing power by increasing the blood flow, oxygenating the cancer cells and tissues, and sweating out toxins.

Nobel prize winner Dr. Otto Warburg, in an often

duplicated experiment, showed how he could convert normal cells into cancer cells by simply depriving them of oxygen.

As a side-effect of exercise, you will soon have a knock-out figure. You will look and feel your very best. A store of energy will be released that will enable you to work more efficiently at your career or job; or, if you are sick, that your body can use to recreate wellness. You will soon radiate renewed and refreshed revitalization. You can count on your body responding to the encouragement of a vigorous, regular workout.

My prevention of recurrence routine now divides into half weights and machines and half swimming. With this program, I hope to build such a resistance to breast disease that I never have lump problems again. So far, six years later, so good.

Exercise has to be combined with a low-fat, high-fiber, low-protein diet such as the MOTEP diet (See Chapter 7) in order to create health. It is not enough to exercise in the morning and then go to lunch at a fast food drive-through and order a double cheeseburger, french fries, and a large, thick milkshake. You may be nulifying your efforts.

In one scientific study, two groups of rats were observed.[18] One group was fed a high fat diet and put on a

---

[18] Thenneson, Harry J., Ronan, Anne M., et. al., "Effects of Exercise on the Induction of Mammary Carcinogenesis." "Cancer Research" 48. 2720-2723: May 15, 1989.

treadmill for exercise, while another group was fed a low fat diet and remained sedentary. Both groups were then injected with a carcinogenic substance. To the researchers surprise, the rats on the high fat diet who were exercised on the treadmill every day grew the greater number of breast tumors and had a faster rate of occurrence of multiple tumors. These rats were also heavier due to increased appetite from their exercise routine.

However, on the whole, researchers have found exercise most beneficial. For instance, a study of women who were athletes in college and kept up their exercise were found to have a decreased incidence of cancers of the reproductive system throughout their lifetime.[19]

Another study showed that extensive physical activity inhibited either tumor growth in transplantable tumors or tumor occurrence in chemically induced or spontaneous tumor modes.

The hypothesis of this study was that worked or fatigued muscles may produce a substance that inhibits tumor growth. Drs. Paschkis and Hoffman studied rats with tumors. They found reduced tumor growth and even "spontaneous remissions" occurred when these mice were injected with an extract taken from healthy mice that had just been

[19] Shepard, R.J., "Physical Activity and Cancer." "International Journal of Sports Medicine." 1990: Dec. 11-6 413-20.

exercised to the point of exhaustion.[20]

Habitually worked muscles are stronger and more flexible than flabby ones and are better able to resist invasion and erosion by opportunistic cancerous cells.

As well as becoming stronger, a well exercised pectoral muscle can also better resist tumor attachment (the first place a breast tumor will attach itself is to the skin in front and the muscle behind).

James Ewing, an early cancer researcher (1920) found the highest rate of occurrence of malignancy among the physically inactive. He also did a study of eighty-six thousand cancer patients which revealed the highest death rates of those that did the least exercise.

In the Simontons' book *Getting Well Again,* the authors state: "We began paying more attention to exercise when we discovered that many of our patients with the most dramatic recoveries from cancer were physically very active."

They mention as reasons: release of stress and tension through physical activity, and changing one's state of mind, was well as a way the patients can participate in their own healing.

Aerobic exercise in which you pant and/or sweat has further benefits in that it stimulates the immune system, revitalizes the organs, increases blood blow, increases

---

[20] Hoffman, S.A. and Hoffman, K.E., Pashikis, et. al., "The Influence of Exercise on the Growth of Transplanted Rat Tumors." "Cancer Patient" 22 (1962) 597-99.

metabolic rate so that toxins are eliminated faster, oxygenates the blood, and lowers the fat content of the body. There is a direct relationship between oxygen uptake and performance of physical activity.

Why is this oxygenation of the body so important? Normal cells in the body divide by mitosis, that is they split exactly in half. They have forty-six chromosomes which divide into two cells with twenty-three chromosomes apiece. These cells need and thrive on oxygen. However, cancer cells, according to Dr. Gerson, cannot divide normally. Often they have too many chromosomes. They don't divide but instead multiply by fermentation. This is defined by the dictionary as ``a chemical decomposition of an organic substance by a chemical agent.'' According to Linus Pauling, tumor cells release an enzyme hyaluronidase which allows these cancerous cells to proliferate and eat through barriers placed in their path such as normal healthy cells and tissues. Normal structures simply fall apart as their cementing ground substance is attacked by this enzyme. The tumor grows and thrives living off the normal tissue's food while the patient becomes more and more emaciated.

However, cancer cells, unlike normal cells, abhor oxygen. That they simply cannot live and proliferate in a highly oxygenated environment was demonstrated to me at the cancer convention where they projected a slide of a cancer patient lying in an oxygenated ``space capsule.''

This is one alternative way to treat cancer. The high dose of oxygen kills the cancer cells.

This high-tech apparatus may not be readily available to you, but an hour of high-energy, all-out aerobic exercise **is.** Oxygen uptake and delivery *must* match the demand of working muscles.

To make sure you are working hard enough, check your pulse rate during and after exercising for fifteen to twenty minutes. You can find your pulse by putting two fingers closest to your thumb at the top of your neck roughly halfway between your ear and your chin. The following is a target chart:

AGE	BEATS PER MINUTE
20	150
30	140
40	130
50	120
60	110
70	100

Count the number of beats you feel in a six second period and multiply by ten to get the minute rate.

For me, hard, physical exercise was a way to take back control of my body, to revive a weakened immune system, to reinvigorate and revitalize, to spend an hour away from all my worries, to rejuvenate and become rebirthed, to shed debilitated tissue and deteriorated cells and replace them with healthy, full-blooded ones. It was a way to inform my body that I meant business; I was going to get rid of my lump and get well.

Every morning in the enveloping liquid which afforded me both resistance and pleasure, I conveyed this message to my body. I also like to "sing" when I blow bubbles which bothers some of the other swimmers no end, but to me was very therapeutic and soothing. You might try this, but expect some commentary.

Exercise also improves posture. Posture is connected to self-esteem. Practice standing and walking very upright with chest out and shoulders down. Slumping and holding tensions within creates "blocked" areas that may become stagnant. Oxygen-deprived cells may then become starved thus, perhaps, becoming cancerous. This is a theory of mine based on the fact that when I feel anxious and fearful, I hunch up my body and become tense. I did just this for a year before the lumps were found in fulcrum-points of that tensed position.

Just for a moment tense up your body and fold it within while you are seated. Perhaps you can feel what I did to my body. Even when I drive, if I begin to think of negative things or have bad feelings, I can now feel myself sliding that tension down to my left hip. Catching myself, I now can relax and release that tension. In my studio, I would hunch my shoulders forward worrying about the recession. That tension ended up in the inner portion of my breast.

Exercise releases that tension block, oxygen cleanses it. When you exercise, chemicals such as endorphins, "nature's high" are released creating an over-all feeling of pleasure, energy, and well-being. Stress simply evaporates and is replaced by calm confidence, energy, and strength. Time is allowed for an inner-strengthening with no distractions from this journey.

At the same time I had the lump in my breast, I had a pain in my lower back. This was probably from the tumor in my uterus as it grew pressing against my internal organs. This pain disappeared at the same time the breast lump dissolved. My general decline into an unhealthy condition, stressed-out with lumps and pains was gradually changed into vibrant health through the hard work of work-outs.

Do not expect overnight success if you are ill. It took time to get sick; it's going to take lots of time to reverse that direction toward wellness. Yet exercise is the compass to point the body in just that direction. Your vigorous routine will signal the body that health is around the corner. Dead, destructive, and immature cells are going to be replaced with healthy, fully oxygenated ones. Every day working hard toward this goal, you will regain strength bit by bit, cell by cell. You will slowly regain health. The threat of emaciation from cell theives that steal your strength will be replaced by the toughness of newly built-up muscle tissue resilient to inroads by destructive enzymes. A pallid, or yellow palor, will be replaced gradually by a rose-hued glow, skin bathed in highly oxygenated blood and toxins sweated out.

Part of my routine was to take a sauna before and after my swim. One alternative cure for cancer is found in subjecting the body to another disease which creates a fever which heats the body and also kills the cancer cells. At the end of the nineteenth century, William B. Coley, a surgeon, was frustrated when he found surgery was futile in the treatment of his cancer patients. He noted that one patient had recovered from life-threatening bone cancer when he suffered a skin infection that gave him a fever. He experimented, injecting patients with live bacteria which he called "Coley's Toxins" which produced a fever. These patients suddenly underwent "spontaneous regression" of their tumors.

A similar condition may be experienced by our bodies when we raise our bodily temperature by sitting in a hot sauna until we sweat. Without injecting ourselves with Coley's Toxins or catching malaria, we may be helping our bodies rid themselves of cancer cells or tumors by heating and sweating them out.

Coley claimed forty-one percent cures in sarcoma, cancer of the bone and connective tissue, by using this method. In breast cancer, very impressive results were also achieved. (R. Moss p. 123). Using fever as a therapeutic tool is an idea that dates back to Hippocrates.

Rather than getting sick to get well, I substituted the sauna. My body soon responded with its own fever—the inflammatory reaction I described which then began to obliterate the tumor. This may be all theoretical on my part, but the fact is—it worked. Three weeks after this red-hot feverish reaction in which my breast turned into burning stone, the rock in my breast completely dissolved, the pain in my back disappeared and no tumors have returned. Healthy cells gradually took over completely.

"What should I say about exercise?" I asked Kimberly when I visited her in the hospital while she was undergoing her bone marrow transplant. She had just finished five days of intense heavy-duty toxic chemotherapy when I steeled myself and boldly walked into her room to visit her. I experienced the shock of my life!

Nothing prepares you for the devastation of the human body intense chemotherapy leaves in its wake. A concentration camp victim of neuter sex stared back at me. Her head was bald except for a stubble of brown, her face pale and lifeless, her eyes sunken in.

"Physical strength builds mental strength," she said through gritted teeth in a voice that seemed to come from some far off tunnel deep within her.

I nodded, trying to stay coherent. Maybe if I interviewed her for my book, I wouldn't break down and sob in front of this shell of a creature that used to be my gorgeous, honey-blonde feminine friend.

"In a few days I will have absolutely no immune system. It will be zero!" she wailed.

"You look much better than I expected," I gulped, trying to sound convincing.

"I can't even drink two glasses of orange juice without getting sick," she muttered.

"Linus Pauling says chemotherapy breaks down the gastrointestinal lining, the villa that digests food," I noted. "But I'm sure you will get over that soon."

"Gerry misses me," she sadly intoned, the saddest I had yet heard. "When he comes to my room, he lays here in bed with me."

"I called Gerry. . . he seemed very upset and emotionally drained and exhausted from this ordeal you are going through," I confirmed about her husband. Tears were beginning to well up and I was trying hard not to break down myself. This was becoming a more and more impossible task.

"Is all the cancer gone?" I inquired, a rhetorical question as I knew from my research that chemotherapy had proven mostly ineffectual in cases of breast and lung cancer.

"No. There is still some left. We'll know more in forty-five days. They give me a lot of tests." She paused as I was very silent. "You don't believe in chemotherapy, do you?"

I was trying very hard to be supportive. But I couldn't lie.

Facts are facts. I slowly shook my head.

"I have to sleep," she whispered and turned onto her side laying in a fetal position.

I turned to go. All of a sudden she shot bolt upright as if on a spring, a corpse come to life in some macabre horror film, as if propelled by some huge effort of self-will. I could see she wanted a hug. I grabbed her and she held on very tight. How could so much strength be left in her?

"I love you Susan," she said.

"I love you too, Kimberly. Get well!"

The spectre of this medically neutered and poisoned phantom of my friend continued to haunt me the rest of the evening. They had taken away her breast, burned her skin, poisoned her, removed her hair, given her arthritis throughout her joints with a silicone gel breast implant, and robbed her of her immune system, femininity, and ability to drink orange juice, not to mention three hundred thousand dollars, all in the name of "treatment!"

I had tried going to a local Chamber of Commerce meeting that night. A glass merchant had invited me. But all I could do was get some orange juice (sympathy thirst?) and go out and stare at the sky which was composed that evening of steel-gray clouds from which seeped out a burnished red light in a blaze of dying sun. I saw this dramatic, changing sunset through eyes glazed with tears not even trying to fight them back.

Chemotherapy is wrong, I thought. It's a crime! How can a poison which takes away her immune system, the only natural defense she has and turns her into this prisoner-of-war be called a medicine? It seemed to me that all this so-called treatment, from the mastectomy on, was some form of violence against women. Male cancer patients, too, were subjected to most brutal, barbaric treatments.

Hippocrates had admonished to future physicians: "Above all, do no harm." This is in the oath all physicians take upon graduation from medical school. How could they rationalize subjecting this beautiful woman to these harsh procedures?

Kimberly and I were both exercise devotees. We met, actually, at the gym. (Remember, exercise is only one factor in prevention. Kimberly's diet was, at the time, what I jokingly referred to as "teenage"—hamburgers, french fries, and large ice cream sundaes). We were both also under a lot of stress and had unresolved psychological problems.

Kimberly did not trust her six-mile hikes which had managed to cut her breast-cancer-now-lung-cancer down by one-third. She thought she needed something "outside herself" to rid her body of cancer and opted for this six week experimental bone marrow transplant. As we soon found out, this gruelling procedure did not effect her lung cancer in any way—the number of cancer cells stayed exactly the same.

I believed the cure for my breast and uterine disease was within myself. Exercise would be a major part of my self-healing process. Perhaps with all her hiking and a bit more patience, Kimberly would have eventually gotten well on her own. She had quit her high-stress job and spent her time resting and exercising. She changed her diet and looked quite good before going into the hospital submitting her body to this transplant.

But now we'll never know. Will she get well because of/despite the chemotherapy? She is still young, she is still strong. I pray for the miracle to happen.

The next week when I call she is already back on the bicycle for half-an-hour per day and eating some solid food. Exercise has gotten her through three years of this disease and three years of treatment (which is worse?). A skeleton of her former self, she is yet alive. She is back on the bicycle! Her stamina and courage are miraculous. She is already rebounding!

Meanwhile, I throw myself into my life, my art, and now my writing growing healthier every day and getting my strength from my exercise program. I have faith that whatever happens, my body—with the proper positive encouragement—can totally heal itself. I pray every day for Kimberly. Perhaps, by some miracle, she will still continue to live.

Faith, Determination, and Visualization; How To Turn On The Healing Power of The Mind

11

"PULL OUT THE FORCE!" Donna gestures as if yanking out healing power from deep within her body. She is a jovial woman seemingly always about to burst into smiles and laughter. We are seated at a Buddhist meeting where she occupies a leadership position. "The Cure for Cancer resides within us; we have the power to heal any illness."

Donna loves her job as a school psychologist where she works with abused and latch-key children. Her spiritual practice is an important tool for her. She utilizes it everyday for self-growth, daily problems, and self-healing.

Life had not always been so joyful for Donna. In 1973 she was diagnosed with rapidly spreading ovarian cancer. At this time in her life, she had accumulated more stress points than most people collect over a lifetime. During the *same* two-month period she suffered these traumas: first, her husband ran off with another woman. As her career depended upon this partnership (she sang in a duet with him creating six record albums), she also lost her career. Along with her career went her income. At the same time her mother was in the hospital dying of ovarian cancer. Her life had suddenly turned into a living Hell. Her health broke down with the illness for which she had a genetic propensity.

Surgery was recommended and it was done immediately to no avail. Her ovaries were removed. Still the cancer returned. Next her cervix and uterus were removed. Still the cancer recurred in the long, empty space where her organs used to be.

About this time she met a Buddhist at a job she had found to temporarily support herself. This woman taught her how to chant. She began to throw herself into the practice, chanting Nam Myoho Renge Kyo in front of a scroll (Gohonzon) which represented her life. She decided to abandon her job and chant for seven hours a day for six days straight. While she chanted she used an aggressive visualization. She imaged little lions eating her cancer cells. At other times she envisioned a cleansing light pouring through her body as she chanted, sometimes through tears. Still another visualization she used during those six crucial days was to aim an arrow and shoot this weapon at her cancer cells.

After the first day of chanting she decided this was

"good medicine." She slept refreshed and well for the first time in months. She continued to chant. After the sixth day of this all-out devotion to a Spiritual Power greater than herself (the Universe), finding the humility to seek help, and making the strong determination to heal herself; she felt well. She had an intuition, strongly felt, that her all-out effort had paid off in complete self-healing.

She went back to the doctor who tried in vain to find any trace of cancer. He was so shocked he sent her to another doctor to no avail. Four doctors failed to find *any* cancer. Since 1975, she has been in complete remission and has had no trace of the cancer which once threatened her life.

"Physical diseases are manifestations of spiritual diseases," Marius, an alternative healer explained. "The mind is the subject, the body the object. If you believe you can get better and take responsiblity, you will get well."

I totally agreed with Marius whom I met at the Cancer Convention. The first thing I did when Doctor Furr found the lump in my breast and the one in my uterus, yelling at me to see a surgeon and get a biopsy, was to decide I was **totally responsible** for my own health. Buddhism is based on cause-and-effect. The sum causes of all your efforts in life is called your karma. If you are ill, what are the "causes" you made in your life to surrender your health? What "causes" did you make to get into a life-threatening situation where your body is deteriorating?

"You have to work backwards," Diedre Morgan advises. "You have to change the chemistry of your body."

What had I done to get my system into this situation?

Reviewing my stress-filled life, the feelings of panic, anxiety, and hopelessness I had experienced the previous year, a path of change opened for me.

"You got yourself into this situation. Only you can get yourself out," Buddhism seemed to be saying to me. If the determination is there, if the faith is unswerving in your own curative powers, in time with lots of work the deterioration of your body, the lumps and pains, will be replaced by vibrant health and a feeling of total well-being.

When chanting for something, in Buddhism, the prayer is based on "expectation" that whatever you are chanting for will happen. The basis is not blind faith or hope. You *expect* to receive whatever you are praying for.

"You had faith." David said upon hearing what I had accomplished. "You had a fighting spirit," my friend Irene added.

In Buddhism you get what you are chanting for because of both the "causes" you make (you think of many ways to help others and help yourself while you are chanting) and the "mystic law" which somehow operates independently to give you "luck."

Whatever spiritual practice you select, its importance

cannot be overstated. By nature we are spiritual beings, even though we are born in a material form. Our energy is tied to the spiritual and when this vibration is blocked or ignored, we suffer.

When we as a culture abandoned faith and religion, we lost a valuable healing tool. Hospitals are now sterile environments whose basis is science, machines, and tests. We've totally forgotten that Hippocrates was a priest; his "hospital" a temple. Healing wasn't a scientific, mechanical process of drugs and surgery, but rather a place where spiritual healing could take place assisted by mineral water hot springs, vegetable soup, and temple sleep with interpretation of dreams. He taught that when our health begins to fail, we may derive profound spiritual benefit from the struggle to regain it.

"You can't sleep in a hospital," Kimberly said to me. "They are always coming into the room to fix something or do something. At six in the morning they change my I.V.s! I wake up every time they come in here." She finally had to resort to putting more drugs into her body, sleeping pills, in order to sleep. "When I get out of here I am going completely off any pills or drugs," she vowed. Unfortunately, she was unable to keep this vow.

I've come to visit her. Her description of her treatment by the hospital staff reminds me of the description of a hospital patient by Lawrence LeShan as "a disease which somehow has a person attached to it."

She now is sitting up and looks somewhat better. She still has a very old, tired look. She now has no immune system and no hair. She runs a fever occasionally from any infection that comes along.

I've decided to chant for her. I begin chanting, after she has agreed, through the surgical mask I've had to wear in order to enter her room in the bone marrow transplant unit.

When I finish she comments, "You look funny chanting with that mask on."

This critical observation (she even laughs) tells me she can't yet get down to that spiritual place. However weird I look, the spiritual feeling I was trying to convey was, I felt, still there.

"It's a feeling," I try to explain. "When you enter the spiritual, transcendent place, you will feel transformed."

I vow to try again the next time I visit her. And the next time I meet with more success. She is now seated outside on the lawn in the sun and resembles a Buddhist monk with her hairless head and simple white garment. She even *looks* spiritual. I tell her Donna's story. She then agrees to chant with me.

The Mormons and the Seventh-Day Adventists have the lowest breast cancer rate in the United States. What do they do differently? Besides being vegetarians, the Seventh-Day Adventists are a close-knit community who gather together regularly to pray and practice spiritual activities. They support each other in all ways and even help each other financially. The basis of their life is their faith.

The Mormons eat meat. However, they don't drink or smoke. Their life is based on their faith and communal activities. Group spiritual activities, praying, singing, and helping others through their home visitations and missionary work is the basis of their life. They devote themselves to a Higher Power: they are able to humble themselves before God. Abstaining from "worldly desires" is stressed. Instead, values of courage, honesty, loyalty, and trustworthiness are emphasized. Faith, devotion, and family orientation are the way of life. The Mormons are close-knit and community oriented. Devotion to worship, spiritual activities, and the giving of a ten-percent tithe describes the lifestyle of the Mormons. They depend on faith and prayer in order to get them through life. They stay healthy, somehow avoiding the high breast cancer rates experienced by their American sisters who are, on the whole, not religious or spiritually oriented.

What is the reason that another spiritual group, the Jewish people of America, are high-risk for breast cancer as contrasted with the Mormon's low risk? The Jewish diet is Eastern European and fairly rich with chicken-fat (schmaltz), cheese blintzes with butter, cream cheese, and sour cream. Still, is the Jewish diet that much fattier than the

Mormon diet which is typically American for the most part? One theory might be that the Mormon women seem to be happy with their roles as wives and mothers (they have a "Relief Society" to go to when they get tired of it and want a break), but some Jewish women are often frustrated with this role. Often they long for an intellectual or creative life. The role of wife and mother makes them "chafe at the bit." They feel "tied down" and dissatisfied. Perhaps this frustration, if not fulfilled by an outlet, begins to chip away at their health. It couldn't be all genetics, could it? Although research scientist Mary-Claire King is on the fast-track of finding the culprit gene (it is located in chromosome 17q), this information might help us only if we had perfect internal X-ray vision and could say, "O.K. Seventeen, shape up!"

In the meantime, what can we learn from all this that will help us avoid or heal breast cancer?

Setting a goal of incorporating a spiritual practice into your life of prayer, meditation or chanting twice a day for even five minutes or better yet, twenty minutes will serve as a protective factor against breast cancer. Joining a group that meets once a week to chant or pray together also seems to have a therapeutic and preventative effect. If you are currently fighting breast cancer or want to prevent recurrence, a spiritual practice is the key to mental and physical health. Buddhists believe that the mind and body are one: shiki-shin funi, two but not two. They believe faith can prevent and cure disease. Their literature is full of examples which they call showing "actual proof"—people overcoming chronic illnesses through chanting and helping others in their practice of faith.

If you simply can't get into spirituality or religion, the next best practice you can acquire is meditation. To me, meditation is not as good as it lacks the essential spiritual component and is too passive. But when combined with visualization, it has proven highly effective in reversing cancer as well as being an aid to prevention.

To illustrate how to do a cancer reversing meditation, let's listen to the guru of visualization, O. Carl Simonton, as he instructs breast cancer patient Jill Ireland when she visits him as she describes in her book, *Life Wish* (p. 64).

"Relax yourself. Physically relax yourself. I'd like you to focus on your breathing saying "IN" as you breathe in and "OUT" as you breathe out. Being able to relax in the face of fear is incredibly powerful and very healthful. Now relax once more, deep relaxation. Now let's very simply go into thinking about cancer, moving very gently into that, specifically focusing upon the cancer cell being a weak, confused, deformed cell. And as it takes energy to push that belief in that direction, make a fist right now and think about cancer being a weak disease composed of weak, deformed cells and relax your fist.

Now think about your body's white blood cells. This is your representation, really, of you— and begin to think about your white blood cells doing the job they're intending to do. Just as the wave does what it is intended to do, what it has done for millions of years, your white blood cells are doing what they have been programmed to do, what is built into them to do. You need to supply them with energy, so you think about them going around taking care of the body. I want you to appreciate that and think about them. If they see any cancer cells, they destroy them. It's that simple because that is what they're built to do, and you make a fist at this point, giving them energy. They need energy. And so you're giving them the energy to do what they know how to do. You don't need to teach them anything. You need to supply them with some good energy. Think about them going along doing their job very competently, very potently, then just relax your fist.

And now, think about your life going in the direction you want it to go. Just the idea and the universe helping you, helping your life. You don't have to figure it out. You do what makes sense to you and open yourself to help. The wave doesn't sit around trying to figure it out. You don't need to figure out the direction of your life. You do what you understand to do, and you open yourself to help. The universe wants you to be healthy. The universe wants you to be happy. You open yourself to help, and the help will come; and that's something you need to practice. Merely by opening yourself to help and asking for it and waiting for it as you do what you understand to do."

Jill felt, after coming out of this meditation, "as if a dark cloud had been vacuumed away from my head." When she first visits him he asks her about her life. She describes how busy she is doing things for her houses, family, friends, and animals, using caffeine and pain-killers to keep up the pace and quite simply, not taking care of herself.

Simonton doesn't mince words, "I'm telling you, you are living a very unhealthful lifestyle. If you don't change it and start honoring yourself and taking care of yourself and taking care of your needs, you will die."

Jill fought her battle courageously and gives us an account rich in detail and humor. But in the end her lifestyle was something she could not or would not change. The tragic death of her son was the final stress she could not handle. She died in her early fifties of a recurrence despite orthodox medical supplemented with alternative treatments.

Meditation, prayer, chanting, and visualization are tools we can use in our everyday life to disperse the stresses and anxieties of contemporary existence. We live in a fast-paced high-anxiety world often filled with danger. One way we can cope without breaking down into ill health is to devote ourselves to a spiritual or meditative practice.

"I would be floundering if I did not have a connection to God and His protection and love," said Eleanore, a Mormon neighbor. "I would feel lonely, alienated, and lost."

The Buddhists believe that chanting to the Gohonzon offers them protection as they are connected to the rhythm of the universe.

When we meditate, pray, or chant for a period of time, our brain-waves slow down to what is called an alpha-wave state. In hypnosis, a trance-state is achieved by relaxation that is comparable to the transitional condition we are in just prior to falling asleep. The relaxed brain is highly susceptible to suggestion. We can suddenly quit smoking, lose weight, or get well by programming our subconscious in this relaxed "open" state.

In the meditative state our blood pressure lowers, the acid-alkalinity of our body changes and becomes balanced.

Max Gerson found many of his cancer patients also exhibited a blood-pressure abnormality—usually too high. A meditative practice can lower the blood pressure back to normal.

At the Cancer Convention, Geronimo Rubio and Bill Fry

of the American Metabolic Institute, an alternative cancer hospital in Tijuana, Mexico, reported that ninety-five percent of their cancer patients had a PH level that was overly acidic. You can test your PH Level by using litmus paper, PH testing strips, on your urine sample. Your PH level is like the ocean tides and goes up and down throughout the day. The ideal condition is to achieve a balance. Meditation, prayer, and chanting, as a daily activity helps us to accomplish this homeostasis, this balance.

The big reward of regular meditative/prayer/chanting activity is the release of stress as we learn to focus our minds on either our breathing, a scroll, or God, and away from our everyday problems and worries.

According to Dr. James Privitera, another alternative cancer researcher, stress is the number one cause of cancer. He stated that stress increases adrenalin production within the body that makes platelets stick together and puts out "growth factor" which supresses the immune system. We know Michael Landon complained of a blood clot in his leg right before the doctors found he had pancreatic/liver cancer, from which he died. The doctors told him there was no connection between the blood clot and his cancer. According to Dean Ornish, in his book *Dr. Dean Ornish's Program for Reversing Heart Disease,* blood clots during the "fight or flight" response to conserve blood in case the threat is invasive and might cause the person to bleed to death.

This might be a new avenue for cancer research. According to Dr. Privitera, we should look to the blood as to who shows excess clotting to predict both heart attacks and cancer. He recommends blood thinners: heperin, niacin, fish oils, garlic oil, vitamin B-6, bromamine, magnesium, ginger, ginseng, and primrose oil.

Prayer is another route to stress release and balancing the chemistry of the blood. When practiced regularly, anxiety and tensions melt away drowned in brain-released endorphins.

I have gout and cannot digest fats because I am missing an enzyme. I have to avoid both excess fats and stress. Under stress my body manufactures too much uretic acid which has the same effect as if I overate a highly fatty food such as shrimp. The end result is an overly acidic blood condition which results in a gout attack in which my body throws out calcium "stones" into my joints. Many early breast lumps found by mammogram machines turn out to be calcium deposits which may or may not become breast cancer. There is some connection here. The only substance which "turns off" my gout attack is colchicine, derived from the Autumnal Crocus which is not a drug, but has been known since Roman times to stop gout attacks. This small pill seems to "thin" my blood and calm it. The attack abates and my body stops throwing out calcium stones. These stones, I have found, do not need to be surgically removed.

Though they are extremely painful in the joints, they finally go away after some time if the stress is resolved. I had two gout attacks when I was under heavy-duty financial stress early in my career as an artist. Since I have learned to control my stress level through chanting, I have not had any attacks, nor have I had to take any colchicine or other medication to avoid them.

In Buddhism there are ten worlds. These worlds reside within us. *Hell* is not a place we go after we die, after living a life of sin, but a "life-condition" we experience presently here on earth. It is a state of extreme suffering dominated by the impulse to destroy oneself and everything else. The second lowest "life-condition" is *Hunger*—a state in which one is controlled by desires for fame, wealth, pleasure, power, etc. and is never truly satisfied. The third lowest "life-condition" is *Animality*—a state governed by instinct, in which one has no sense of reason or morality. There is a tendency to take advantage of those weaker and resent those who are stronger. The fourth lowest is *Anger*—a condition dominated by a selfish ego. One who is compelled to be superior to others in all things has this life-condition.

Upper worlds include *Humanity, Heaven, Learning, Realization, Bohisattva,* and *Buddahood*. These states include controlling desires, exercising judgement, and observing morality and ethics and being able to maintain **tranquil human relationships.** Rapturous joy, even if short-lived, seeking the truth, compassion for the suffering of others, and desiring happiness for others and finally Buddhahood—a state of oneness with the ultimate truth, the True Self, absolute freedom, boundless wisdom, and infinite compassion comprise the upper spheres of life conditions.

All day we go up and down within these ten worlds. We might go to Heaven when we receive a check we have been waiting for in the mail or Hell when we suspect our mate is having an affair. Our life, then, has both positive and negative aspects. It constantly changes from moment to moment. Through spiritual practice, it is possible to gain the wisdom and power necessary to raise our life-condition up from the lower states. We chant to be able to attain an "unshakable high-life condition" so that we are not rocked around as much by life's ups and downs.

Hell is the lowest of the Ten Worlds and is called jigoku in Japanese. The character for "ji" literally means "the earth or bottom" while the character for "goku" literally means imprisoned, tied down, or loss of freedom. In other words Hell is a state of life in which people suffer and can do nothing about it. They can't escape. They suffer every moment. In the world of Hell, people have no power to influence the environment, no hope for the future, and are incessantly suffering either physically, spiritually, or both.

Hell is full of anger or indignation as well as pain. Nichiren Daishonin, the Eastern sage of Buddhism states,

"Rage is a state of Hell." In our daily lives, if we fall into despair over our circumstances and are controlled by our suffering and agony, then we are living in the world of Hell.

It is constantly living in this state of Hell, a living death, which causes our immune systems to break down. This low-life condition gives cancer cells the opportunity to grow and start to take over, in my opinion

In this over-stressed condition, the will to live is simply not strong enough or predominant. We don't care if we live or die. We may actually wish we were dead. In an interesting scientific experiment, a group of terminally ill cancer patients were asked under hypnosis if they wished to live. Seventy percent said no!

The mind is the best medicine cabinet. By learning to control the mind through a meditative or trance-like state, we can learn to raise our life-condition. We can focus on becoming happy. We can chant or pray to help others and extend ourselves out to others. Making others happy will go far in increasing our own happiness and health.

The ultimate goal is to become happy.

Happy people do not get cancer. This seems to be the Golden Rule that runs throughout the scientific, medical literature. Learning chanting, meditation, or acquiring a prayer ritual each day will help us to maintain health and happiness.

In the medical literature, Dr. Max Cutler cites a seventy-eight year old woman with breast cancer who lived on for ten years without surgery, radiation, or chemotherapy (she refused medical treatment). She was a religious fanatic who had developed (what the medical community called) "a strong paranoid reaction," shortly after the onset of cancer. She "didn't need treatment because God was saving her." She was vituperative in the expression of rages. "What role could this character structure have played in her miraculous span of life with cancer?" he wonders.

He also found a small group of people who seemed to be able to live on despite their cancer. "They all have the same calm, peaceful appearance and demeanor and I have often sensed them looking at me with astonishment as to my concern for them. This small group of patients that did well seemed to have a very special attitude: an overwhelming faith that **all is well and will continue to be well.**"

His most striking example, a patient with widespread cancer of the breast metastasizing to the supra clavicular and cervical lymph nodes following radical mastectomy, has continued in remarkably good health and spirits. When questioned about the degree of apprehension or anxiety which she experienced on being told of the diagnosis nine years ago, she expressed amazement at the question, assuring me she knew she would be perfectly well because "the stars told me so."

IN OTHER WORDS, IT WAS HER ATTITUDE RATHER THAN THE

SURGERY THAT KEPT THIS WOMAN ALIVE! WHILE SURGERY DID NOT STOP THE SPREAD OF HER CANCER, HER FAITH KEPT HER HEALTHY ENOUGH TO KEEP LIVING.

Here is a Buddhist speaking who is also a doctor: Dr. Chris Lawrence of Seattle, Washington, a neurologist:

"Some of the illnesses (of my patients) stem from simple things such as poor posture, inadequate exercise, or poor methods of dealing with stress. These would correspond to some of the physical causes of illness. No matter how far the medical science develops, there will always be the need for the Buddhist practice to change the karmic causes of illness.

I really appreciate my Buddhist practice as I chant daily for the wisdom and compassion to make the right decisions for my patients. There is still a lot of art in medicine and this is the part that is developed best by Daimoku (chanting). As President Ikeda mentioned at the twelfth annual SGI meeting, "It is in an individual's behavior that the essence of Buddhism lies."

In my case, I had no idea that my own health had deteriorated under the stress of my Hell life-condition until Dr. Furr found the lump in my breast and began his four-alarm campaign to get me to the surgeon. By chanting, I was able to conjure up the life-force, the will to live, and the determination to change my hopeless, deteriorating life-condition to one of radiant health and happiness. I was able to make drastic changes in my life, "causes" that would point my life in the direction of health. I quietly and without anger (I have that characteristic of cancer patients—trouble expressing negative feelings) extricated myself from a relationship that held no future and was rapidly turning me into a co-dependent always waiting for my turn to see a man who was becoming more and more distant. I wrenched myself away from an emotional relationship with him, turned him into a friend and went on with my life. I was able to ask one of my wealthy collectors for some financial aid. He was happy to help me as he could see me suffering through the recession. I dusted off my writing skills. I began to see the suffering and anxiety I had endured were actually a "benefit" since I could share with other women how my single-minded determination to turn my condition around eradicated a breast and uterine tumor without surgery.

My self-centered artist life revolving primarily around me, myself, and I had brought on illness and attracted other self-centered people into my life. When I began thinking of others and how to help them, my life changed. My friend Marlene dragged me to a singles event where, kicking and screaming and only wanting to leave immediately, I met a loving, kind, and generous man who brings me flowers and takes me on trips.

When I stopped abusing myself, I attracted a different sort of person—one that wouldn't abuse me. The Buddhists say, when you change, your environment changes.

When I raised my life-condition through chanting and prayer, I was able to stop the self-destruction that was ruining my life. I was able to get out of Hell. I slowly walked the pathway to health. The tumors gave up, went away, and stayed away. My debilitated condition slowly and steadily became one of vibrant health.

An important part of the MOTEP program then is single and group spiritual activity. Incorporating faith into your daily life whether it is religion, meditation, or prayer will help you to avoid breast cancer. If you should find a lump, a spiritual practice is one element of the program that will help you rid yourself of it.

"What is the most important thing you did?" I have been asked by women either trying to reverse their breast cancer themselves or trying to get well in conjunction with medical treatment.

"I had a deadline. Set a deadline and work everyday through prayer and visualization to get rid of your cancer by that date. When are you going to be well and free of all cancer?" I ask them. I listen as they set a date. I then see a different person. I see a changed expression on their face—one of determination. I see a person with spiritual conviction and strength who at first looked more like a confused and frightened victim.

This is the most important part of the MOTEP program—

the spiritual expectation that you believe you will get well in two months, or whatever deadline you set. For prevention it is the spiritual conviction that you will stay well. You are protected by the Universe, God, or a Higher Power. If you fall ill, you will be able to rally and unleash your own powerful healing forces with the faith that you will soon get back to vibrant health.

Stress— Give Yourself A Break! 12

A shroud of mystery surrounds the subject of breast cancer. Fear, anxiety, and frustration accompany any conversation on the subject. It is a black secret we are somehow ashamed of. And yet the subject is now coming out into the open.

"Breast cancer has increased twenty-four percent since 1974," announced Diane Feinstein at an election party campaign. She was running for U.S. Senator, a race which would prove victorious. She would like to see more funds for research appropriated to fight the disease. As for the rapid increase of this modern epidemic, she can only ask, "Why?"

Fran Visco, formerly a breast cancer patient, now in remission, has started "The National Breast Cancer Coalition," a grassroots advocacy effort. The brochure she sends out begins with this bleak cover item: "In the time it takes to read this brochure, another woman in this country will be told she has breast cancer." The last page presents this hopeless information: "There is no cure for breast cancer. There is no known cause." She would like congress to appropriate three hundred million dollars for breast cancer research. This group successfully lobbied Congress and persuaded it to double the amount of money it spends on breast cancer research ($133 million to $197 million).

However, spending tremendous amounts of money trying to find an external cure has not, in the long history of cancer, resulted in any clear answers or remedies. Paradoxically, the harder we look **"out there"** for the "cure for cancer" the less chance we have of finding it!

It is time to look within.

"When I think about my sister I feel a heaviness in my chest," Nan, a beautiful woman in her forties gestures as she describes how she holds in the tension and sorrow she feels when thinking about her sister, who has had a second re-currence of breast cancer. Her mother died of the disease in her forties. Spontaneously, she has revealed an important piece of information that may have dire implications for *her* future health: where she carries and stores the grief and distress she feels about her sister's situation. Is this a family trait? Is the total responsibility for this family disease all due to genetics? She explains the difficulty of having any kind of relationship with her sister who lives in another state and with whom she can't get along. Their relationship has always been difficult and distant. When I talked to her a few months later, her sister had died. It was too late to mend the relationship.

If Nan could have communicated her sorrow and distress to her sister instead of tensing her upper torso with the burden and storing her distress internally where it may fester, she would have, perhaps, helped to save her sister, as well as healing her own life of emotional pain. Now, any chance to convey her feelings was lost.

If we look to the possible external causes of breast cancer or reasons for its alarming escalation, we can find any number of possible suspects. Yet not everyone exposed to carcinogens, which are impossible to avoid in our modern environment, develops cancer. This fact must lead to the conclusion that the onslaught of external stresses which we all face everyday of our lives are still not as important as how we internalize them.

Certainly a case could be made for the breast cancer epidemic to be totally iatrogenic in origin, pointing the finger at mammograms, birth control pills and implantations, and estrogen replacement therapy, which exude hormones and steroids. As estrogens are chemical messengers, what horrendous stresses are involved in giving the body the information in the form of birth control pills that it is pregnant when it is not? What about the stress of duplicity in tell ing the body through estrogen replacement therapy that it's still fertile when it's trying to do its normal work of shutting down into the retirement of infertility? Anytime we try to lie, manipulate, or confuse the body, we upset the balance and invite illness.

In the newest shift in research, scientists are now targeting hormones instead of fat as the culprit in breast cancer. Has anyone noticed that taking exogenous hormones for the purpose of birth control or staving off the effects of aging has been firmly nixed as a remedy for **men?** Steroids have been firmly banned for athletes as they can cause horrendous physical damage such as loss of limbs! Yet we let physicians talk us into putting estradiol patches for menopausal symptoms on our rear ends. Estradiol is a steroid! With hardly a second thought, we implant birth control (Norplant) in the arms of young women who may become breast cancer patients twenty years down the line.

As to external pathogens, our bodies are able to mount what Norman Cousins refers to as a "prodigious response" to the challenge of bacteria, viruses, mutant cells, and disease. However, our immune systems and healing systems do have trouble when we are under long-term stress. This seems to be the over-riding factor that tips the scales toward disease.

What exactly is stress? And how does it contribute to lumps in the breast?

The concept of stress was invented by Hans Selye who distinguishes between *stress* and *distress*. While stress is ever-present in our daily life, distress is what takes its toll on our health. He points out that the everyday stress we experience is not harmful, but is rather what he calls the "spice of life," and very necessary for our growth as human beings. This was illustrated to me by my college friend, Jackie. She is a brilliant woman who loved foreign languages, art history classes, and literature. But she had conflicting goals. On the one hand she wanted to travel, especially to Europe, to study art, mingle with writers, and perhaps write. Her father was an interior decorator who loved working with richly pat-terned fabrics and wallpapers. She worked with him in her spare time and developed an eye for exciting interiors.

On the other hand, she confided to me one evening that she just wanted to find a rich man to marry. This way she would avoid the stressful aspects an independent life might entail.

She soon found her rich husband, a contractor who built up-scale tract houses. As he loved to build, he would no sooner complete one project than he would be off to a different state to start yet another. Jackie moved so often that she soon gave up any attempt at interior decoration. She had a child and spent her time in one empty house after another. Her dreams of foreign travel and mingling with artists gave way to living in various new bare white-walled homes.

When I visited her I was shocked by the emptiness of her house. There was no art on the walls or even carpets on the floor. It seemed to me she had given up many of her interests and dreams and lived an empty life in a vacuous environment.

She later wrote that the doctor told her she had a disease with a very long name. When I looked up this strange-sounding affliction in a medical reference book, I was not very surprised to find that this disease was often the result of leading a very boring life!

At age 51 she developed breast cancer.

Clearly, stress itself is not bad for us. It is, in fact, a necessity for us to keep our health: "Bored to death" is an expression that holds a bit of medical truth. We could call it **"the stress of avoiding stress."**

Lawrence LeShan spent his career with cancer patients whom he felt would fit into just this category. In his book, *Cancer as a Turning Point,* he describes several cases of breast cancer in which the women had given up their dreams in order to pursue a life of self-sacrifice to others.

Maria, for instance, a physician who supported her poet husband and twin daughters while doing work she disliked, and lived in a city she was not comfortable in so her daughters could receive a special education, developed a lump in her breast at age forty-eight which she ignored for a year until it had metastisized beyond the point of surgery being an option.

LeShan, a psychologist specializing in cancer patients, talked with her for an hour. He writes:

"She saw no possibility of work that she would enjoy, of living where she would like to, or of a life that would make her glad and excited to get out of bed in the morning. Her husband and children were very happy with their lives and she was successful enough to allow them to continue it.

"Rather brutally, because I felt I had to shock her into taking action on her own behalf, I asked her how she planned to continue supporting them in the style to which they had grown accustomed after she was in the cemetery as her cancer prognosis was so poor. She looked completely defeated.

"After a long pause, she said 'I know I can't do it anymore. I had hoped that you would know a road for me.' Her sadness and despair moved me deeply, and for a few minutes we both just sat there."

When she decides to take charge of her life, assign her family part-time jobs, and splits the housework, making a career change to a position she enjoys and taking summer vacations to South America, her home, her tumor shrinks and stabilizes and four years later she is still alive and enjoying the fact that she finally took charge of her own life and redirected it toward her own enjoyment and fulfillment.

In another poignant case, LeShan tells of how one breast cancer patient rejected his help. In confronting this patient, he asked if he had done something wrong. She replied that she could see where the therapy was going—it would eventually force her to confront the problems in her marriage. She feared this would cause her to lose it. If she had to make that choice, she told him, she would rather choose death. Which she did.

Perhaps if she had thought ahead, I mused after reading this bleak account, she would have realized that in losing her life, she would **automatically** lose her marriage!

In LeShan's view, the "stress" that most threatens our health and opens us up to cancer is not noise pollution, or the everyday stress of solving our problems and overcoming obstacles at home and at work. It is despair.

> "This despair was so deep and hopeless in most the people I saw that there was fairly little emotion connected to it. There was no rage or pain—it was part of their world and had always been there as long as they remembered it."

These patients went on with their lives, maintaining routine while not believeing that life would hold any real satisfaction or meaning for them. Their lives lacked self-expression, self-fulfillment.

LeShan quotes W.H. Auden's definition of cancer, "Foiled

creative fire."

When LeShan worked with these people, digging to help them find "their song," and supporting them in their effort to sing it, he often had miraculous results in "curing" their cancer.

If we take into account LeShan's views, which certainly sustain credibility, we must count in the oppression of women in our society, the road blocks put up in their path to fulfilling their goals, as one of the causitive factors in breast cancer. Until society changes, coming up with child-care facilities, more flexible work hours, and equal pay for equal work, equal opportunity and acknowledgment for their contributions, women will be frustrated and suffer, sometimes to the point of illness.

Now that we know how the "stress of avoiding stress" works its damage on us, let's go back and look at stress itself.

Any major change in your life causes stress. The scale of life-change called "Change Units" was devised by Drs. Tom Holmes and Richard Rahe and is used to tally points in a person's stress life. While points are given for such changes as moving or getting fired, the big "Life Event Changes" that score the heavy-duty points are EMOTIONAL, EMOTIONAL, EMOTIONAL.

Death of a spouse is number one, divorce is second, and marital separation third. Next on the list is a jail term! Sitting behind bars is still not as bad as losing a spouse.

While a healthy body is well-equipped to handle short-term stress, **chronic long-term distress** is what breaks down the body into a diseased state. The body reacts in a stereotypical way to any exacting demand made upon it.

Hans Selye described this reaction in 1936 as the G.A.S. (General Adaptation Syndrome) which had three stages: (1) alarm reaction, (2) stage of resistance, and (3) stage of exhaustion. The adrenal glands produced adrenaline. The thymus gland, located in the chest, the master immune gland that works with the lymph nodes, shrank (the lymph nodes themselves also shrank). Then gastrointestinal ulcers appeared.

It is very interesting to note that Selye produced this reaction in rats when he forcefully immobilized them, or once, when experimenting for another reason, he injected them with extracts from the ovaries! Since the ovaries are the main producers of estrogen, this shows a definite link between excess estrogen and stress. Excess estrogen in the body, then, could easily lead to disease.

The body increases its supply of hormones in order to be ready for the "fight or flight" response it has been called upon to make. The fearful stimulus has caused an emergency response. The body has prepared you to deal with the threat quickly so that you can protect yourself and go on with your life. However, *if the fearful threat continues over an extended period of time,* **even if only imagined,** the excess adrenaline, noradrenaline, cortisol, and other hormones and steroids will cause the body to break down at its weakest link. For women, especially as we get older, this weak link target organ is the breast which is also the target organ for estrogen.

A vigorous immune system will catch mutant tumor cells and immediately destroy them. T-cells actually squirt a poison into the cancer cells, B-cells destroy tumor cells, machrophages vacuum up odd cells, and natural killer cells do battle with mutant cells. If the body is under stress, however, the number of natural-killer cells actually decreases, the lymphphocytes disappear; mutant cells are then free to multiply and form a tumor. Other defenses of the body are still called into play. The tumor is cordoned off with a protein coating (thus the rock in the breast). Interferon, interleukin, and tumor-necrosis factor are used as weapons. If the body is detoxified and strengthened it can use inflammation to isolate the tumor and cytokines, rapidly moving and buzzing like angry bees, to attack the tumor.

However, all these weapons of the body cannot do their job if we remain tense with distress. There is a good chance they will lose their battle if we are not able to induce in ourselves a feeling of calmness, and well-being.

To better understand the new field of psychoneuro-immunology or how the mind talks to the nervous system, a must-read is Kenneth R. Pelletier, *Mind as Healer, Mind as Slayer.* He describes the technical connection between emotion and stress: (p. 52-3).

> "There are two primary physiological systems which are activated by stress. One is the autonomic or involuntary nervous system, and the other is the endocrine system (hormones). It is at this point that the role of the hypothalamus in the midbrain becomes increasingly important. This unassuming structure seems to exert decisive control over both the autonomic and endocrine systems. The hypothalamus is closely connected with the brain's limbic structures which are related to emotional behavior."

Cortical hormones are so potent that when left in the body for long periods of time, they can do irreparable damage to the kidneys. (Cortisol is also a steroid.) These adrenal hormones were designed for *short-term fight-or-flight reaction only.* Only one drop can change our rate of heart-beat, metabolism, or body temperature!

A constant communication takes place between the brain and the immune system. Immune cells such as lymphocytes have neuro-transmitters and neuro-receivers by which they relay messages to and from the brain. The immune system has a nervous system!

This exciting new information explains why, when doctors tell a cancer patient that they are terminally ill and have only two years to live, they often die right on schedule. Conversely, relaying a positive message as I did, that I absolutely must get rid of two tumors in two months, resulted in my immune system responding to meet the deadline. This news is vital for doctors treating cancer patients. The negative or positive message they convey to their patients becomes a self-fulfilling prophecy.

Seven years after prolonged financial stress, Diane Hinton discovered she had ovarian cancer when her doctor had her submit to surgery for a grapefruit-sized tumor in her abdomen. She and her husband had been mired in debt because of financial losses during the 1982 recession when they had lost their cafe. They recovered financially, but Diane became ill. The article about her in the "Los Angeles Times Magazine" (October 20, 1991) does not link up the stress she went through over an extended period of time to her illness. Instead it focuses on a dramatic new treatment being tested at UCLA by a physician-scientist team headed by Dennis Slamon. After surgery (a hysterectomy and several tumor removals) and two rounds of chemotherapy over a period of months failed to stop her cancer (the tumors increased in numbers), Diane is turning to this new experimental gene treatment which involves monclonal antibodies taken from mice who churned out this substance when injected with oncogenes similar to what Diane's tumor has: Her-2 neu gene which codes for the production of a growth-factor receptor.

The antibody zeros in and attaches itself to the gene in the tumor cells in a lock-and-key fashion to reduce tumor growth. This treatment is entirely new and experimental and has yet to show any therapeutic value in humans, though it has reduced tumor growth in mice. It is currently being experimented with at UCLA on ten patients with ovarian cancer and ten with breast cancer.

We already explored Dr. James Privatera's view that under stress the blood is supplied with an excessive amount of growth factor which causes the blood to clot and feeds tumor growth.

Tumors, we have seen then, are dependent for their growth and actually have receptors for either a hormone such as estrogen or growth factor, both of which are increased in our blood because of long-term chronic stress. This stress can be emotional, financial, physical, or the stress of one or more major life changes that make excessive demands on the body's reserves. Even a stressful event that is positive can wreak havoc on the body. A rare case of a groom dying at his wedding is an example.

Diane may benefit from this new innovative treatment. Then again, since this technique is as yet unproven she might do as well by learning to de-stress her body, detoxify her body, and employ other self-healing methods such as those outlined in the MOTEP program. She might do some honest soul-searching to find out how she participated in her own disease, to find the CAUSE. Modern medicine based on science and looking for miracle cures ignores both causes and self-healing abilities in its single-minded search for that **magic pill.** But all healing is self-healing: *it must come from within.*

Technology is wonderful. This new genetic engineering technique sounds promising. But the fact is our brain is still better than any computer, and our healing mechanisms, if supported properly and given a chance, can outperform any surgical, drug, radiation, or gene-wonder technique.

Our cells can only be a mirror of ourselves, our life events and how we handle them. If we feel desperate and hopeless, if our life is constantly chaotic and out-of-control, if our daily mental state is characterized by extreme anxiety, depression, pessimism, gloom, and doubt, how can we expect our cells to be calm and healthy and reproduce in an orderly fashion? When we tense up our bodies with fear and negative thoughts and our breathing becomes shallow, our cells will not receive the oxygen they need and they will not have the room they need to move. Innundated with stress chemicals, they become blocked and the result may be a tumor. The organism is beginning to choose death over life.

When the stressor excites the hypothalamus at the base of the skull, it alerts the pituitary gland which in turn regulates adrenocortical activity. The adrenal cortex produces ACTH (adrenocorticothrophic hormone) and releases this hormone into the blood. This induces the adrenal glands located above the kidney to produce adrenaline. Adrenaline is a highly potent chemical designed to give us extra strength in an emergency but is dangerous in high amounts over a long-term.

It is interesting to note that testing for adrenaline in the blood is an accepted method for diagnosing depression. Recently the test has included ACTH. An initial response to fear and rage may, in the long run, turn into depression. This long-term depression, with its subsequent pouring into the body of various strong chemicals designed for short-term use, endangers us and opens us up as candidates for various diseases such as cancer. Another is the common cold.

A recent study reported in the "British Journal of Medical Psychology" related that life events and mood states were of greater importance in the catching of colds than viruses or wet, cold weather.

In other scientific studies, yoked mice injected with tumor cells suffered earlier tumor appearance and exaggeration of tumor size, whereas *escapable* shock had no such effects. Mice left to swim in a deep vat of water died quickly while ones taken out of the vat at intervals continued to survive. This indicates that animals can take extreme stress if they do not feel hopeless or helpless about their situation; if they have some control over it.

When we are depressed, natural killer cells actually decrease. Patients reporting depressive fatigue-like symptoms and who complained about lack of family support, tended to show a decrease in natural killer cell activity levels in one three-month follow-up study. Breast cancer patients scoring in the "risk" range of measures of fatigue, depression, and social support perception could be identified (via killer-cell count) as biologically vulnerable.

This report also notes that **passive patients fare worse** and this fact has been in the clinical lore for decades.

Kiecolt-Glaser demonstrated the enhancement of natural killer activity in elderly subjects trained in the technique of relaxation.

Investigators at the National Cancer Institute found variance of activity of natural killer cells in fifty-one percent of the patients on the basis of three "distress" factors:

1. Patients who were rated as "adjusted" (i.e. passive, stoic).
2. Patients who complained about lack of social support in their family environments.
3. Patients who were listless and apathetic.

Levenson and Bemis found that bereavement as a psychological response to the loss of a relationship alters aspects of the immune function. Immuno-suppressed rodents develop tumors. Humans who are immuno-suppressed can develop tumors at multiple sites and this can happen when they are either under stress or deep depression.

A large body of scientific literature links shorter survival in patients with depressed, resigning characteristics compared to patients who were able to express more negative emotions such as anger.

In a report by Greer, et. al., breast cancer patients who demonstrated a "fighting spirit" or who used denial had a higher survival rate than those with stoic acceptance or expressed hopelessness or helplessness.

Clearly, then, the link between chronic long-term stress and depression to breast cancer and breast tumors is well defined in the medical literature. Long-term chronic stress and depression lowers our natural killer cell activity, allows tumors to grow and floods our system with the chemicals these tumors feed and grow from.

Even before reading all this medical literature, I was able to size up my situation as one of severe stress. My body was tense with it, my sleep disturbed by it. My first assignment in the task of tumor eradication was de-stressing my body. This took positive action.

I began a group therapy monthly meeting. I decided no matter how much stress I was under or what bad news my life situation seemed to be dealing me, *I was not going* to take it out on my body. I simply and firmly separated my extremely stressful situation from myself and held it "out there" at some distance (I couldn't just get rid of it until circumstances in my life changed—and they did change after my resolution). **I forcefully induced a feeling of well-being** even if it took an imaginary hypodermic needle!

Here are some STRESS-BUSTERS you can use to prevent and fight breast cancer:

1. Periodically examine your life. Are you doing what you always wanted to do? If you feel you are frustrated, bored, or unhappy with your present occupation, what steps can you take toward a new direction? Self-sacrifice may seem attractive at first, but in the long-run the feelings it engenders can stress your body to the point of illness.

2. Are your relationships healthy and supportive? Being around negative or depressed people can drag you down. Everyone has relationship problems at one time or another but constant problems in which you just can't seem to get what you need may mean it is time to end the relationship and move on.

3. After a major emotional trauma get into therapy. We are vulnerable to major illness or death after we lose a spouse, go through a divorce, or separate from a long-term relationship. We may think we can handle it, but the facts show otherwise. Getting into group or individual therapy for a year or two after a major stress has occurred in our life

can save it. Doing something active and positive when under stress such as expressing grief, or sharing problems with others who have been through similar experiences, can help us get through a rough period in our lives with our health intact and our breasts devoid of tumors.

4. Get into an exercise routine. A one-hour-a-day five-to-six-days-a-week vigorous exercise routine will help "burn-off" excess anxiety and stress, increase the blood flow, and generally aid us in both health and disposition.

5. Get plenty of restorative sleep. "My machine works long hours without getting tired. All I need is four hours of sleep a night," said Michael Landon just before he died of pancreatic/liver cancer.

6. Don't be a complete loner. We all need other people, even artistic types like me. Admit you have needs and plan your life to include other people. The more love you give out, the more you will receive.

7. Make it a point to laugh. When we take life a little less seriously and can laugh at our own foibles, we take a large step toward de-stressing our body. **Just try laughing at the same time you hold your body in a tense, closed anxious way.**

8. Incorporate a period of time each morning and evening for meditation, or chanting, or prayer. (Even if for only five minutes.)

9. Recogize when you are depressed, when you have

bitten off more than you can chew or when your life isn't working. This is the time you are most likely to be vulnerable to breast cancer and other diseases. Work on reversing that depression by taking positive steps toward change: reaching out to others, spiritual activity, group therapy, asking for financial help, finding a new relationship, taking courses in the field you really wanted to work in, taking mini-vacations so you don't succumb to workaholism. Be assertive about your needs; they are most important!

As an exercise when I feel depressed I think of wonderful things I have. I begin with the phrase, "I'm lucky. . .and go through ten advantages out loud. For instance, "I'm lucky I'm alive!"

Daisaku Ikeda said, "If you do nothing but fret and sigh because of a setback on one front of life, this can end up bringing your whole life down in defeat.

A defeat is rather the time to build up your energies; you must make defeat the stepping-off point for the victories that will follow.

Being able to do this is the secret of life."

The Cancer Personality: Changing Poison Into Medicine **13**

Upon sitting down to rest on a Yoga mat at the Cancer Convention, I inadvertently met Joy. She was describing a dream about her third metastases of breast cancer which now lodged in her shoulders and neck. I couldn't help eavesdropping when I heard, "a big, beautiful animal on my shoulder, gorgeous! Looks like a loveable puppy; a bridge I made myself composed of warm fuzzies."

I did a quick double-take. Joy was a beautiful, vibrant, golden-haired woman who was describing an insidious, vicious and life-threatening disease in terms of something she not only welcomed, but actually seemed to be fond of and proud; even loved! I was horrified, at first. My instinctive reaction was avoidance but curiosity got the upper hand. I had to know the story of this youthful looking woman who turned out to be aged fifty. I asked if I might interview her for my book.

She turned out to be a very friendly, if distraught, woman in very good physical shape. She agreed to do the interview between demonstrations of various Yoga positions on the mats she was selling, some of which involved headstand-like positions. Obviously, exercise was not an element that was missing from her life. What was?

During the interview in which she talked about her life, her eyes welled with tears of sadness. "I have an addiction to not thinking well enough of myself," she admitted.

The history of her breast cancer went as follows: at age forty-five she had had a lumpectomy for a breast tumor. At that time she also went to Mexico for cleansing, diet, massage, and vitamin supplement treatments. She was then fine for two years. However, the tumor reappeared at the incision site after that time. She also had a satellite tumor. Her next step was undergoing more surgery, this time a quadrantectomy, a pie-shaped removal of a portion of her breast.

"Last year was psychologically bad and emotionally devastating," she recounted. "I worked too much and was careless about my diet. That's when the cancer returned in my shoulder and neck."

After the surgery and chemotherapy her attitude changed. She realized there was no "magic bullet" that would rid her of the cancer. She had to pay attention to where her vital energy was blocked. She now was into phase four cancer which was considered by the doctors as not curable but controllable. She began doing "Inner Child" work based on the writings of John Bradshaw. She realized she was a co-dependent. She had more energy than she could use, so she "stuffed her energy." Also she deprived her body. Her tumors disappeared when she let go of sadness and resentment "from people who have hurt me" but recurred when she continued hurtful relationships with emotionally abusive men who used her.

She described her current boyfriend with whom she has gone for seven years. "The man doesn't want to grow up, doesn't want to commit, doesn't respect me or accept me as I am."

She lived with him for two years, helping him remodel a house he had bought. When they were finished doing all the work he told her, "I don't want anyone sick around here; I don't want anyone old and ugly." She then moved out, renting a small room in a large house which she describes as "too small."

She continues to see him once a week. I told her I was in a similar co-dependent relationship when Dr. Furr found a lump in my breast. Part of my recovery was breaking off this relationship, or rather turning it into a friendship which avoided emotional abuse. I advised her to do the same. But she refused to even consider the idea. For some reason she seemed to need and want an abusive relationship. Several times she spoke of "beating myself up." She had decided to remain with the man despite her description of him as never having had any wives, of being "emotionally screwed up" but always having women around as co-dependents. "He's using me," she admitted. "He knows how to use women."

However he wasn't the first man who used Joy. Her husband, by whom she had two sons, had also treated her badly. After her divorce she met a charming man, a body-worker whom she put through chiropractic school. However, he couldn't get a job upon graduation and subsequently left her. She lost her home from the accumulated debt of putting him through school. She described herself as being in pain for two years after that experience. "RESENTMENT WILL KILL YOU." She further stated, "The price you pay for being resentful is you get to do yourself in."

As I shared this woman's tears and pain, I couldn't help feeling that she was somehow rewarding herself with her suffering; that she needed or thought she deserved self-destructive situations in her life and depended upon them to feed a feeling of low self-worth. How could I get her to see this?

Her problems originated in her childhood where she was the oldest of four children. "Dad gave us all a hard time. But I took it too personally, too hard. I was always trying to get his approval. His attitude was that I was never good enough. He never was appreciative."

Her current boyfriend was a reflection of what she called her "poisonous family," as he too continually told her she wasn't good enough, rich enough, or tall enough. She called this man "the best thing in my life."

"Happiness is the root of all health," she explained to me through her tears.

I began to feel a responsibility to "get through" to Joy whose very name began to sound ironic. The next day she gave me that chance.

"What was the most important thing you learned in this conference?" she asked me.

I told her it wasn't something I learned in the conference. The most important thing I had learned in my self-lumpectomy program was to set a deadline as to when I would rid myself of the tumor. In my case, Dr. Furr had set the deadline. To him the date meant a follow-up exam with further brow-beating to try to get me to see a surgeon. To me, however, this was a target date I used as a goal to get well.

"When are you going to get rid of all your cancer?" I asked her point blank.

She thought a moment and seemed conflicted about making a decision but finally picked "the Ides of March." I was surprised she picked a date that was so far off, since it was now only the beginning of September. Was this a reluctance or postponement on her part for getting well? Did she have reasons, however subconscious, for wanting to stay sick? Perhaps pity was the one way she had found in her life to obtain the love she needed. Perhaps there was a reason why she had internalized her resentment about the way her boyfriend treated her. Was this cancer a substitute for having to express her feelings of anger toward him, a physical "accusation" against him? Was the cancer a mute protest, an imprisoned pantomime of her wrath? Whatever her reason, she definitely had one for holding on to her cancer, for postponing any major effort to get well.

However, after she had picked the date, I was surprised a little later to see a "new Joy." The blithe, carefree facade, the careless attitude about her disease which came out when she spoke of visualizing her cancer "being broken up into Tinker-Bell sprinkles" was now replaced by a fierce attitude of determination. She had turned a facade of flippancy and false gaity into a "woman who means business" attitude. Perhaps she was on the road to health. Maybe she could now see a reason to trade in her "raw deals" and self-destructive urges for the will to live.

"You do good work," she told me later.

I am not a therapist; I'm an artist. Yet in order to rid myself of my own breast lump, I found it necessary to do a lot of work on myself and also to go into group therapy. I, too, was "beating myself up." I, too, had very critical, punitive parents I found it impossible to please as a child. But, unlike Joy, I simply had no desire to hang on to destructive urges. When the physical proof of ill health showed up in my body, two tumors, I was able to put my self-destructive urges into hand-on reverse. In order to do that, I had to first **"make the determination."** I had to live in the "here and now," as psychologist Fritz Perls used to say. I had to see my life as it was. I told myself, I'm willing to make any change. I'll change *anything* in my life in order to get well. This was the most important first step. I then began a systematic divesting of anything that might be hurting me or contributing to the downhill course of my health. Step-by-conscious-step I began trading the urge for self-destruction into the will to live.

My life wasn't working. If it were I would not have this piece of granite in my breast. That was the bottom-line conclusion I had come to. My body was suffering. If the man I was seeing was dragging me down into frustration, jealousy and loneliness; I would take a hard line, admit I was hanging on to nothing, and find another man more responsive to my emotional needs. If the recession with its bleak financial picture eroded my strength in day-to-day worries about how to pay my bills, I would ask for help. I am so stubborn about making it on my own as an artist that asking for help is, to me, almost an admission of defeat.

Yet the fact was, I needed help to make it through the

terrible recession bordering on depression which the United States was going through. The "trickle-down" effect was more a description of my state of health at the moment than an economic policy conjured up by Ronald Reagan in the hopes that helping the rich would somehow, in a convoluted way, bolster the situation of the poor and the middle-class. It hadn't worked. The rich had slowed or stopped their purchases of art.

If research showed I had more chance to get rid of a lump if I chose a semi-vegetarian diet and under-ate, then much as I loved meat I would discipline myself with a new diet. If exercise would help me, I would throw myself into a vigorous program of getting up early and swimming a mile. Visualization had once proven effective for me; then a program of chanting and visualization must be set up. Psychologically, I needed help so I sought out a group therapy meeting. The willingness to change and grow and to discipline myself was the beginning of the self-healing program. With words and action I informed my body that it was time to get well. I began an interior journey, looking within for the strength to transform myself.

Dr. Frederick B. Levenson, in his book *The Causes and Prevention of Cancer,* theorizes that all cancer begins in infanthood.

Babies waving their arms and legs are discharging tension from the irritation they are experiencing. If the mother is unable to respond to the infant's cry for help due to loveless conditioning she had in her own earlier life or an unsupportive husband, the baby learns to hold this irritation within.

Dr. Levenson states that he has seen a basic trait in all his cancer patients: "She will have developed all sorts of emotional defenses to prevent herself from being unconditionally loved and accepted. She will be uncomfortable, embarrassed, and sometimes even appear provoked if love is directed at her."

If her emotional needs are not met as an infant and she learns to be self-contained, to hold feelings in, and to see life as a basically irritating experience, she may be vulnerable to cancer in later life. We know that cancer is caused by irritation whether it is an external carcinogenic substance or internal carcinogens of excess stress hormones or other bodily chemicals which cannot be expelled from the body in time to prevent damage to the cells. When we hold onto stress or negative feelings, adverse chemical changes in the body may lead to uncontrolled cell growth.

Jill Ireland describes just such a childhood in her book *Life Wish* (p. 74). With her therapist, she regressed in memory "to the despair and grief I felt as a baby of ten months when I had Pinkus disease and was left in the hospital for some months in a glass incubator in isolation." When her mother visited her she would cry and hold out her arms to her, but her mother was not allowed to hold her. Finally her mother decided the visits upset the baby too much and stopped coming.

Michael Landon describes his mother as "mentally ill." She made several dramatic attempts to commit suicide. "When I started high school, my self-esteem was in the gutter," he related.

Gilda Radner writes with her right hand, "Is this cancer my mother inside of me?" Her left hand answers, "She doesn't want me to exist." Gilda filled the hollow, loveless void with chain smoking and overeating leading to Bulimia.

We see in the case of Joy how she consistently managed to play the role of victim. Repeatedly she gave while asking nothing in return. "Being taken" by others, continually abusing herself and her body, intent on proving her worthlessness and unloveability to herself and those around her seemed an unconscious goal. Apparent is her fear of relating to others in a healthy give-and-take way. It was almost, in her relationships, as if she were asking men to abuse or take advantage of her.

Despite her impressive ability to articulate her problems, her capability to actually face them and to institute genuine change seemed almost non-existent.

In asking Joy to set a deadline in which she would rid herself of all cancer, I attempted to give her hope. When I suggested she could have total control over her body in order to **will** herself well, her whole attitude changed. With this new hope and determination, she may very well cure her "incurable" cancer.

Norman Cousins describes a woman who was able to rid herself of a life-threatening breast tumor after he told her she could use her mind to "program" herself. What he was referring to, actually, were the good results she could expect from surgery. She had balked and refused surgery explaining that she thought surgeons were "too casual" when it came to amputating women's breasts. After teaching her biofeedback techniques in which she raised the temperature of her hands by visualizing the blood flowing to her extremities, she went home and signed up for the surgery. However, she must have experimented with "programming" and applied it to her breast tumor because when it came time for her to go into the hospital, her lump was gone and her breast was once more soft and supple. Cousins describes being speechless at this result. But he had taught her something brand new, he taught her **control.** When she found out she could use her mind to control her body, she must have experimented with this new knowledge to learn "self-lumpectomy." She used her mind to heal herself, thus avoiding surgery which she did not believe would help her. "Self-lumpectomy" was not a concept in Norman Cousins' mind. Certainly, the medical profession has not used this terminology in any text book. In fact when Cousins looked up "healing system" in the medical textbooks, reference books, and even medical curriculums, he could find nothing. Medical knowledge and systems are built upon diagnosis, procedures, and treatments. Other than the immune system, there is a vacant space where knowledge of how the body rebuilds and repairs itself should be. Actual experience has taught me that "self-lumpectomy" is not only quite possible (I have done it several times), but may be intrinsic to getting well.

A childhood which was marked by feelings of isolation and depression makes us more vulnerable to cancer, especially in a situation where these feelings are allowed to return. A person with this type of childhood must seek relationships in which they feel rewarded, wanted, and needed rather than ignored, frustrated, and thwarted. It is of crucial importance to women with this type of personality to seek out warm, loving individuals as equal in give-and-take as possible. At low points of life, therapy is a valuable tool. Learning to love oneself is a basic component in wellness. Sometimes we need help to learn how to do this.

An isolated childhood led me to go off into a corner to color with my crayons. Instead of becoming autistic, I became artistic. I learned to channel feelings of aloneness and isolation into expression and creativity at a very early age. This way I could be alone and still communicate in a silent way. This tolerance of isolation through inner expression enabled me to be able to spend long hours alone in the studio and even prefer this type of activity to socializing. Many of my art school contemporaries who did well in Art School could not tolerate the loneliness that goes with the long hours of solitude a professional full-time artist must withstand.

However, isolation must be balanced with social relationships, otherwise disease may develop. It was not until much later in life that I discovered a need for people. At first I felt awkward when it came to making friends. I still must work hard at this aspect of my life, as being alone is what seems most comfortable to me.

When Dr. Furr found the stone in my breast, one of the first things I did was seek out a therapy group. Instinctively, I knew a warm, loving group of people with whom I could share my experiences was an essential ingredient in a wellness program.

One evening during our group therapy meeting we decided to add excitement and a change of pace by using Rune cards to predict the future. These illustrated, oversize playing cards are an ancient method of prediction dating back to the Vikings. I approached this pastime with great trepidation as my health situation was extremely questionable at the time. No one in the group realized this. We were to pick two cards apiece.

The first card I chose was a beautiful illustration of two

swans, their long necks lovingly entwined. The explanation on the back was that I would soon have a partner. The single women in the group sighed wistfully and nodded approval.

My next card, however, was a shock! It depicted a glaringly lit hospital operating room with a long, empty table over which a surgeon in a mask, headcovering, and rubber gloves menacingly loomed. The caption was, "The patient on the operating table is you!" The woman later told me I turned white and mute.

The explanation was that I had something in my life that needed excising. The advice was to "operate on yourself!"

I was so very glad to have the support of a friendly, warm group then. The cards offered a confession which I did not have to verbalize. The cards had revealed my problem. The Runes, with their ancient wisdom, knew my secret. I was terrified not only by the message of the card but by its uncanny accuracy. I sat stunned. On the long drive home I chanted, "Operate on yourself!" over and over.

"Vogue" magazine reports in "Mind/Body Medicine" (Sept. 1991) how group therapy is the latest weapon against disease. Dr. David Spiegel at Stanford University found this out inadvertently when he set up a group therapy session for one year for fifty women with metastasized breast cancer. All of them knew they were dying when they began these sessions. Although the study was set up merely to show that group therapy would reduce anxiety and depression and improve coping skills in terminally ill breast cancer patients, the doctor was stunned in a follow-up study (the sessions were conducted in 1977) to find two of the women *survived* and one lived on until 1990!

Compared to those who did not participate, women in group therapy lived twice as long. "Social support seems to be one factor that shows up again and again that seems to influence many different illnesses," says Steven Locke, author of *The Healer Within*.

Spiegel further goes on to say that, "frankly, group support may have a more powerful effect than many of the other physical interventions we do." And he believes that support groups should be part of any treatment for major illness. "Having a support group to share pain, laughter and fears Is a very powerful thing," he states.

In further research he noted that male cancer patients did better If they were married, while women survived longer when they retained strong ties to their **women** friends.

The urge toward self-destruction is often at the root of many diseases which represent a partial suicide, according to Karl Menninger in the book *Man Against Himself.* He ascribes ulterior motives to self-punishment. Unconscious motives include aggression (the will to hurt someone else rebounded on oneself) and an erotic component. He believes this aggression toward someone else backfires because of guilt. Martyrs who turn themselves, however subconsciously, into invalids—or repeat surgery patients—are granted special privileges and even greatness for being able to bear their continual suffering. Self-punishment can also come from the habit of being regularly punished as a child by parents. In this case self-destruction is what we are used to. Martyrs turn others around them into martyrs. A wish to be a sort of "Queen of Suffering" and thus be elevated to a heroic/tragic sphere has been observed in patients with recurrent diseases and operations. In the erotic component, bleak, ordinary suffering is turned into an ecstasy of pain. "Some men and women will go to incredible lengths to submit to cruelty, deriving conscious sexual satisfaction from ill treatment."

That mystic and ecstatic experience come to many through deprivation, degradation, and physical torture in the service of a cause, is well known, according to Menninger. However, while the "orthodox martyr" recognizes his self-sacrifice for a cause, the neurotic invalid denies seeking self-destruction. Since there is no apparent "cause" for this sacrifice, the entire preoccupation seems to be with the self.

This type of martyrdom is unprofitable and wasteful. Whatever satisfaction a person gets out of continual disease and/or hospitalization is certainly not worth the pain involved. Menninger ascribes the substitution of pity for love as due to a sense of guilt arising from powerful but inhibited aggressions. There is a conflict between the wish to live and the wish to die.

Being a victim, becoming ill, and slowly destroying oneself are certainly ways of receiving attention, pity, love, money, or a valid excuse to relax and take off time from work. However, the personality, in sacrificing its healthy self, pays a high price for this attention. When we choose, consciously, not to be a victim, we take the fork in the road toward health. When we choose love over hate in our relationships, we choose wellness. When we give up resentment and hatred toward others, we give up a weapon of lethal self-destruction. When we give up unhealthy self-criticism, putting ourselves down, and feeling generally like a failure, and substitute self-encouragement, pride, and self-support, we will see our health and our lives improve. When we convince ourselves that we deserve success in our life, that our relationships will be good, positive, and loving, and when we work harder in that direction, we will see our lives change for the better. When we give up narcisstic worrying about our own condition and start caring more about others, we will see a general improvement in our own health.

Self-destruction is, in the end, a completely selfish act. Self-reconstruction is, on the other hand, a vital, healthy act of generosity. When we are willing to give ourselves what we need and want, we will be better equipped to help others. In this way we will grow as human beings. And in this way we will stay healthy or get healthy.

According to Dr. Levenson, the major way cancer patients differ from healthy people is in how they relate to others: RELATIONSHIPS ARE THE KEY. Cancer patients aren't always able to relate in a loving give-and-take way. They have trouble with unconditional love.

Pathologist Charles Sims studies biopsied tissue samples from breast tumors to determine if they are malignant. He has pointed out that although cancer cells are slightly larger, with larger nucleii and "hard edges," this isn't a sure way of telling if the patient has cancer. When I asked him what was the best way he said, "RELATIONSHIPS ARE THE KEY." Cancer cells don't relate well to other cells. He mentioned further that they are renegades, outlaws who don't follow the order of normal cells, trample over others, travel anywhere in the system and use and feed off other cells, while destroying the body.

These self-centered, self-destructive cells resemble, perhaps, a self-centered lifestyle or a turning inward pressuring the body with feelings of fear and isolation. Possibly the "me generation"—the "looking out for number one" (while stepping on others)—has played a large part in the steadily increasing rate of cancer. The increasing isolation of people living in large cities with the inability to communicate and share their lives with others may also play a part.

I am much more careful now as to how I treat people.

I view rudeness in myself and others in an entirely new light, as part of a route to distress, possible failure, and disease.

If there is a clue here for us, the prevention of cancer or the reversal of cancer may depend vitally on our staying around positive people, avoiding "users" and depressed, uncommunicative people, and developing our ability to give and receive unconditional love. By practicing giving and receiving love, not holding onto anger and resentment which erodes our health, we can avoid vicious traps of self-destruction. Carcinogens can be external *and internal.* Internal carcinogens can be far more irritating and destructive than external ones.

Dr. O. Carl Simonton, who overcame cancer when he was seventeen and has worked with cancer patients throughout his career, has noted the following traits which make up his "cancer personality" profile:

A great tendency to hold resentment and a marked inability to forgive.

A tendency toward self-pity.

A poor ability to develop and maintain meaningful long-term relationships.

A very poor self-image.

He finds the underlying factor to be "basic rejection."

The ancient physician Galen noted that internalizing, melancholic women were more prone to breast cancer than cheerful ones.

The Buddhists have a saying, "changing poison into medicine" (Hendaku lyaku)—which means turning a painful, irritating, and even deadly, situation into one which is nurturing and helpful. The first step in doing this, according to the Buddhist method, is to stop blaming others for your problems. When we accept responsibility for our own "karma," we know that any bad situation we got into is our own fault because of past "causes" that we ourselves made. Then, and only then, are we in the power position to change the situation. And we must change when we have a chronic illness. There is only one bleak alternative.

The Buddhists believe the mind and the body are one. Feelings of chaos, anxiety, anger, resentment, and hostility, especially when they are repressed, can lead to a disorder of our very cells and disease.

Dr. Max Cutler asks, "What are the factors which trigger the change from cellular *order* to cellular *chaos*? Is the emotional force the finger on the trigger?"

He found cancer patients had a self-sacrificing attitude and a high degree of unresolved dependency in childhood. Almost all women had a pathological relationship with their mothers—they felt extremely obligated to them and had a high degree of self-sacrifice for them. Underlying this attitude was hostility. Few were able to vent their rage. Studying forty patients behaviorally he found:

Masochistic character structure.

Inhibited sexuality.

An unresolved hostile conflict with mother covered over with a facade of pleasantness.

Inhibited Motherhood.

He concludes, "One must consider an internalized self-destructive drive."

Morgens R. Jensen reported in "The Journal of Personality" (June 1987 317-42) that breast cancer spread was associated with a repressive personality style. After studying fifty-two women with a history of breast cancer and thirty-four controls (who had no cancer), he found a reduced expression of negative affect, helplessness/hopelessness, chronic stress and comforting daydreaming in the cancer patients. He also found a propensity to tune out stress. He reports defensiveness and low discrepancy levels between self and ideal-self ratings. Attempts were made to avoid giving any impression of psychological disturbance. He found they gave impoverished descriptions of emotional experience. They failed to pay attention to stress. They almost never felt the urge to tell someone off. They had impaired attention to their inner experience. They had both more self-deception and more "other" deception. They were more likely to report acting in a calm, confident manner and to appear unconcerned about their problems while being colorless and emotionally flat. They were more concerned with appearing nice and attractive rather than solving their problems. They were more likely to present themselves as responsible, conforming and cooperative while holding their feelings inside and trying to impress others as being well-controlled and serious-minded. They exhibited blocking, avoidance, and denial.

Longer survival was associated with patients who have good relationships with others and preserve intimacy with family and friends. They were able to ask for and receive emotional support. Their anger did not alienate others but rather commanded their attention. They refused to let others pull away.

Shorter survival times were noted in women with poor social relations. Those who had experienced early separations from family and repeatedly had mutually destructive relationships with people, often wanted to die.

Weisman and Worden showed evidence that increased emotional stress contributes to short-term survival. They noted patients who lived longer tended to maintain cooperative and mutually responsive relationships. However, cancer patients with death wishes, depression, apathy, and long-standing mutually destructive relationships survived for shorter periods than expected.

"Those who are at war with others are not at peace with themselves," said William Hazlitt. We cannot expect our very being, our very cells to remain in peaceful co-existence if we are continually at war with ourselves and others.

Although all relationships involve love and hate, when the pendulum swings way too far in the realm of hate, it may be time for first aid in the form of therapy. Perhaps, the only solution is to break off the relationship. Loving, supportive people can be found. It just takes time to look.

The best way to attract love is to give it. Persons who are generous with themselves and others will attract generous people who can care and give love rather than selfishly withhold it. Don't be afraid to ask for what you want and need from others. The self-sacrificing woman who gives and gives, asking nothing in return, but at the same time, harboring anger and resentment at the treatment she gets from others, is asking for unhappiness and disease. If, in reveiwing your current life-situation, all you do is complain and/or cry, you are not functioning at optimum health and illness may be lurking in the wings. High anxiety and a chaotic lifestyle may equal out-of-control rapid cell growth.

Learning to nurture, support, and love yourself is the key to maintaining your health. The next step is to reach out to love and nurture others. Any problem can be used as a chance to change your destiny. Even cancer can be a "turning point."

Always work toward happiness. Try to avoid self-abuse. Seek out positive, warm, loving people and work toward authentic relationships with them. Present yourself in a genuine way to others rather than with some fabricated facade which you think will make you more acceptable. Avoid self-pity and self-flagellation. Avoid negative internal dialogues in which you continually argue with others or criticize and find fault with yourself. Make sure you give and also get your fair share in relationships. No one respects a doormat they can use.

If you are filled with anxiety, practice meditation or chanting to calm yourself. Recognize and admit the stress you are under but don't use it against yourself as a weapon of self-destruction. We all have our limitations and it is better to admit them than to get ill trying to accomplish unrealistic goals. Don't repress or deny emotional problems—that won't solve them or make them go away. Admit you have a problem and go to work to solve it. If your life is chaotic turmoil, slow it down. Work toward inner peace however much resolve this may take. Healing is something we must work at everyday. Dealing with all the stresses of life presents a hardship for the body. Even though I am basically an "iron horse," it only took a year or two of high-pressured stress and ignoring my body to make me vulnerable to chronic illness.

It's most important to your health to be good to yourself and others. Love is the ingredient that turns poison into medicine.

The Good News: Prevent and Eliminate Breast Tumors Without Disfiguring and Harmful Surgery, Radiation, or Chemotherapy

14

The healer Anoush opened the door. His dark eyes emitted a magnetic energy that struck me at once.

I had been sent to the Healer by Nance Mitchell, the skin-care specialist. Ostensibly, my mission was to interview him for my book, but I was also extremely curious as I was told he could heal breast lumps with the energy emitted by his body alone. Of course, this seemed incredible to me. Just as most doctors believe that only *they* can get rid of lumps through surgical procedures, I had just as staunch a belief that the only permanent tumor removal resided within the body itself, through its own healing mechanisms. How could he make tumors vanish merely by using bodily energy?

Anoush bade me sit down as he was with a client, a tiny infant girl asleep face down on her mother's lap. I watched an amazing process as I sat across the room. Anoush would circle his straightened arm over the baby without touching the child. The baby lurched up as he ran his energy over her as if jerked by an invisible string. Even across the room I felt a current of energy as if the whole room was plugged into a wall socket. Every once in a while, Anoush would halt his treatment and lash his arm out from the elbow as if recharging it. After several of these thrusts he would resume his circling.

A knocking at the door announced the arrival of the child's father. There was some heated discussion as he strode into the room. I thought I heard the word "tumor" sandwiched in phrases of a foreign language and a fierce refusal to go with something, some treatment proposed by UCLA.

After they had left, Anoush explained to me that the infant girl had a kidney tumor. It was his art, he said, to be able to heal tumors and make them disappear.

I was still skeptical. Even considering myself an extremely open person who believes strongly in mystical experience, I felt only extreme doubt. Was he serious?

I told him about the lump in my breast which I had gotten rid of myself a couple of months ago. He told me he had healed "hundreds of lumps, some very large." He asked me where my lump had been located.

"You find it," I challenged, deciding at once to test

him out.

He bade me to stand up. Using his arm again, this time as a diagnstic tool, he waved it in front of my body, without touching me, in concentric circles. First he went around one breast, then another, and then back again. I was wearing a layered tunic outfit, with a heavy cotton-knit blouse and long sweater. He did not ask me to remove any clothing. Back and forth. Around and around. Finally, he settled miraculously on the exact spot in my left breast where my lump had been!

I was astonished! "How did you know?" I asked.

He replied that this spot was "heavy." He then looked a bit frightened for me and asked if he might do a complete exam. I was too shocked to object. I stood frozen as he circled around my body from top to bottom telling me that my thyroid was "heavy," as was my right ovary and left kidney. He now looked terrified. He seemed to be as incredulous as Dr. Furr had been when he could no longer find the lump.

"You're lucky!" he exclaimed.

"It wasn't luck," I explained to him. "I put myself on a crash health program covering every aspect of my life."

Thinking back to how much effort had gone into this program and how much self-will and utter discipline summoning up the courage and strength each day to continue, made the word "luck" seem a bit insulting. Of course, luck always plays a bit part in any of these types of circumstances. I *was* lucky that Dr. Furr had found my lumps early enough. I *was* lucky I already had self-lumpectomy experience. I was extremely lucky I did not have medical insurance so that submitting myself to three hundred thousand dollars worth of mutilation and poisoning in the form of orthodox medical treatment had not even been an option. It was advantageous in this one circumstance to be an economically deprived, struggling artist. Actually, I had never considered poverty or economic hardship in the beneficial light of "luck" before. Lack of money now seemed to be a curious but definite advantage.

Anoush looked incredulous. It was his turn now. He was convinced of his own healing energy. He had seen the actual proof of his being able to dissolve tumors. But **self-lumpectomy?** This was something new and magical to *him.* I contemplated that there must be many ways of making breast tumors and other bodily tumors disappear, completely unknown to the American Medical Association.

I asked him exactly what he meant by "heavy," the term he used to describe the areas of my body he felt were affected by my illness. He said that he meant "blocked"—the acupuncture meridians were blocked off. The flow of energy within my body had been stuck at certain points resulting in tumors.

I still wasn't sure of what he meant precisely. However,

the areas he described with his arm did seem "heavy," especially the area where the lump in my breast had been. Any stress I was under also seemed to zero in on that one spot. It was to take the next seven months to rid myself of the "blocks" by sticking to the MOTEP program.

When he finished the "exam" I felt refreshed as it I had just been in a spring-water pool. This dose of energy had somehow transformed me. That night I slept like a rock.

He explained to me that he was a physicist living in Armenia when he had had an accident. During a mountain climbing adventure he had taken a very long fall. Recuperating in the hospital, he began to discover that he had healing energy. After his release, he sought to develop this ability further by studying with a healer. He claimed he now could heal other people using his energy field. He could give me any number of actual examples. His own wife, for example, had had a tumor which he had vanquished using his own bodily magnetic energy. Later, Dr. David Clark would give me some new scientific findings to back this: magnetic particles are being discovered within the cells.

I thanked Anoush and took leave. The transcendental experience I had just gone through confirmed a basic fact that I already knew. The lump in my breast was only a symptom, only one sign, of a decline of my whole body. The growth, a tumor on the upper left part of my uterus that my doctor discovered when he did a pelvic exam at the same time perhaps accounted for the lower back pain I had experienced on my left side which had miraculously disappeared when the lump in my breast dissolved. My disease or degeneration involved many vital organs. Merely removing the lumps surgically or even removing my entire breast and giving me a hysterectomy would not have worked—just as amputating the breast had not stopped the cancer Kimberly was still fighting, the cancer that was now situated in her lungs.

Viewing breast cancer as a "localized" disease involving only the breast is a **fallacy.** It is an expensive assumption which women cannot afford to believe at the cost of their very lives. Surgery as a sure-fire cure for breast cancer must be reconsidered, just as blood letting was finally re-thought and eliminated as a cure for disease after too many patients had bled to death. Since less than two-thirds the women receiving mastectomies and adjuvant chemotherapy and radiation survive past five years, why is this destructive form of treatment continued? Women must be informed medical consumers!

As for me, there would be no let-up of the hour-per-day vigorous exercise, the mostly vegetarian whole-grain diet eliminating meat and dairy products, the absolute prohibition of going out with any more abusive men, and staying away from negative people in general. I needed to continue my chanting and visualization rituals twice a day, work harder to eliminate my financial problems, work more on my positive relationships, and help others as much as possible. Negative silent self-commentary had to be nipped in the bud.

I now had a mission: helping to reverse the upward spiral of the rate of breast cancer. Today a woman has twice the chance of encountering the disease as during the forties, when I was born. Reducing the death rate from the insidious disease, warning other women about destructive lifestyle practices, and outlining a natural healing method became a goal.

A year later I visited Dr. Furr for my annual exam. There was no lump nor any recurrence of a lump in either breast. To his surprise, but not to mine, the fibroid or cancerous tumor in the upper left portion of my uterus had also disappeared. It was time to describe the progression of my illness through its various stages. When I began to talk about my dream of my decaying breast, its putrid smell, and about how the next morning the breast had turned a vivid, inflamed red, he was visibly shaken. "Do you think I had breast cancer?" I finally asked him.

"Yes, you had the symptoms."

Up until this very moment, I had never admitted to myself that I might have had cancer. Even though I was high-risk, had two lumps or tumors, and had gone through a terrifying disease process, I had simply never **labeled** it. The fact that I had no biopsy or other scientific "proof" somehow left me off the hook. I could skirt the issue and call what I had done "self-lumpectomy" rather than conquering cancer. This way I avoided confrontation with that hideous word. I avoided looking straight into my own mortality. I could admit to staring down a chronic disease, but a brush with death, the enormity of that kind of battle was beyond my scope.

"Unlucky are those who are diagnosed," Lynn Fraley, a nurse, commented to me some time later. If I had had a diagnosis, would I have had the nerve to defy the medical route and construct my own healing program? I seriously doubt it.

Did I cure myself of cancer? If I did, I had done it all myself utilizing only inexpensive, natural means at home and at the "Y." I did rid myself of two tumors, that was a proven fact.

If I can do it, I thought, why can't other women?

Cancer seemed to be inextricably and intimately tied up with the personality. Certainly, my obstinate character helped. Whether a person succumbs to cancer, or "spontaneously regresses," or even gets well through treatments seemed to be linked to the force of will and the "fighting spirit." Determination, and positive faith, in the body's own healing processes are fundamental. "Healing is a dynamic process of allowing creation itself to flow with its own rhythms," according to visionary communications specialist Michael Glock. To rally all one's own forces takes experience, courage, and tremendous self-confidence. It takes complete dedication.

These character traits began developing for me as a teenager when I was hired as the youngest lifeguard at the new indoor swimming pool. The first lifesaving test I had taken I had flunked, almost drowning in the process. I persevered at my art and a school which once flunked me as a student, later hired me to teach. The first large-scale painting I sold in New York out of the window of a handsome gallery on Madison Avenue was the third attempt to translate an idea. Two other versions were concurrently in the trash can in L.A. My completely "unprotected" life as an artist sans regular salary had created in me an iron strength which, in an emergency, can be brought to bear quickly on almost any situation.

Bob Dylan might sing that as an artist I "never stumble cause I got no place to fall," but the reality is that I've fallen over and over. The difference is, I get back up. Many times I have been at death's door or put my life on the line as an artist. It's nothing out of the ordinary. Breast disease was, for me, a more-or-less routine challenge.

To rebuild my body from a degenerative, diseased state to one of total, vigorous health took me a total of nine months. Noted author Joan Borysenko points out that healing is a "rebirth." With all due respect to my Mother, who did a fine job, I had to totally rebirth and recreate myself.

The "labor pains" I went through, sweating it out each day on my program proved well worth every effort I made. I taught my body how to heal an awesome disease. This lesson will help me prevent recurrence.

Kimberly's personality is in complete opposition to mine. Though strong in many ways, she is more a conformist. Her attitude toward her doctor is to give him control, carte blanche, and to "do what the doctor says." Her attitude toward her cancer is surmised in a recent conversation. "I read all those books three years ago when I was diagnosed with cancer. I know all about fighting and I prefer not to. My stance is I'm going to learn to live with it."

And yet she is interested in what I have accomplished. We go to dinner and she orders fish and vegetables instead of hamburgers and French fries. She wears a stylish wig which suits her and totally hides her bald head. Now two of her rib bones, damaged by the extensive X-ray treatments she received have broken merely from the simple act of breathing. The treacherous bone-marrow transplant which weakened her immune system had not changed the cancer in her lungs in any way. She has exactly the same amount of cancer she had before the transplant. For the first time in our ten-year relationship she mentions death. What would I feel if she were to die?

I emphasize, as dramatically as I can, that I do not want her to die. It is very important to me that you continue to live,

I tell her. I assure her that cancer is reversible. She looks like she is on the road to health. I say a silent prayer right there in the restaurant.

I wonder about the differences that are intrinsic to our personalities, and the absolute glue, in the form of close friendship, that has nevertheless held us together through the years.

As for me, my life has changed in many ways. My struggle as an artist continues during this recession when art sales still lag. However, I now have added a new dimension to my daily life: writing. I have found I really love to write. The topic of breast cancer has gotten this effort so much interest and support. Everyone I turn to has come up with immediate offers of recommendations or help. A wonderful, supportive literary agent showed up seemingly out of the woodwork, along with several publishers anxious to see the completed manuscript.

The flowers on the table are from the new man in my life. He is so kind and considerate, I wonder how I ever managed to date anyone else. Last night he took me to a concert of the blues singer, John Lee Hooker, 72, downtown in an old Spanish auditorium. This was the same day that Dr. Furr gave me the "all clear" and I felt it was a celebration of sorts. As we gazed down at the incredible talent of the elderly black man on the stage who helped invent the blues and influenced many younger artists, I couldn't help thinking of what went behind all those years and all that talent. How many close calls had this man had with various illnesses, tragedies, and disasters? How many years did he live on hope with only his talent, his love of music, and an occasional "gig" to sustain him? How many times was he criticized, rejected, excluded? How many years of poverty did he slog through? What was the story behind this pillar of strength and power? What enabled this slightly frail man as he sat in front of the microphone in a Mexican chair, to be able to captivate his mostly youthful audience as he belted out the blues?

Here I was, at forty-seven, thinking how strong and lucky I was to be able to be alive and well and sitting next to my favorite man, while Hooker was seventy-two and seemed every bit as youthful as the audience to which he sang. I couldn't help thinking about the resilience of the human body when the spirit is carried forward by the love of what it is doing.

George Burns, at ninety-five, relates the story of how someone complained to him, "George, you drink, you smoke, you fool around. What does your doctor say about that?"

"I don't know. He's dead."

George repeats in his books his credo for a long life: **love your work.**

It was an incredible year. Although I've always had

opinions and theories about the treatment of cancer, this was the year I put my life on the line, put all my theories to the supreme test: the test of life itself. What I gained from this experience is a greater knowledge of self-healing and how the body works. There is unbelievable power in this knowledge. I have a new respect for the human body and its great recuperative powers. I know now that given the proper encouragement and environment, the body will strive and succeed to heal itself of almost anything.

I no longer fear breast cancer or any other type of cancer. I have found out for myself that you can truly fight for your life. And win! **The entire pharmacy for healing breast cancer is located inside the human body and its brain.**

What I Learned About Cancer

I've been on a wellness journey. I've also been on a research journey. On these journeys I learned many things. Some of these include:

Emotional stress and distress can cause the body to grow tumors. This can result in death.

During very extreme stress, the organs of the immune system actually shrink in physical size allowing tumor development.

Lumps and tumors in the body can be a sign of a general, overall deterioration of the internal systems.

Repressing anger can create tumors in the body.

Generally, happy people do not get cancer.

There may be no such thing as "localized breast cancer," confined as a disease to only one part of the body.

Before birth control pills were put on the market, they were known to cause breast tumors and other cancer in mice.

After ten years of estrogen replacement therapy, a woman's chance of getting breast cancer rises to nearly one hundred percent.

Silicone used in breast implants is actually an industrial material used in electronic circuit-boards, the aerospace industry, and tile and window caulking.

Eating large quantities of meat on a regular basis may cause cancer, as pancreatic enzymes cannot digest large chunks of meat and fight cancer cells at the same time.

An excess of dairy products in the diet can cause cancer. This has been known for four thousand years.

Eating whole grains helps to eliminate excess estrogen which is linked to breast cancer. This may be better than taking the drug Tamoxifen to prevent breast cancer or recurrence as this drug causes uterine cancer as demonstrated in a recent study.

High body fat content is known to be associated with breast cancer.

Fat cells produce and/or store their own estrogen.

Undereating "revs up" the immune system if this is done for a short period of time.

Overeating on a regular basis opens us up to disease, even cancer.

Over salting our food may cause cancer.

Except for olive oil, oils sold in the grocery store are over-refined and are missing the vital nutrients which have been destroyed through over-heating. (See appendix and John Finnegan's *Fats and Oils—A Consumer's Guide.*)

Religious fanatics get less breast cancer.

Women in third-world countries who have children at a young age, breast-feed, are slender and don't overeat, avoid getting breast cancer.

The FDA and the AMA are continuing their "witch-hunt" after alternative healers—Jimmy Keller who set up a clinic in Mexico and helped heal many people (I've talked to some) is now in jail.

A dentist who wrote a book about alternative treatments for cancer was persecuted by the AMA for "practicing medicine without a license."

Laetrile, the mysterious "alternative drug" is actually vitamin B-17, readily available in twelve hundred different foods (see a partial list in the appendix) and contains natural cyanide which the normal cells use to kill cancer cells.

Over forty years of research by Kanamatsu Sugiura of

Memorial Sloan-Kettering, analyzing laetrile's ability to stop the growth of tumors, stop breast cancer metastasizing to the lungs, and even to prevent breast cancer in laboratory animals, was supressed by the "Cancer Establishment" (NCI and ACS) in order that they may continue to sell chemotherapy drugs.

Vitamin C is a great weapon in treating cancer.

Beta-carotene is converted into Vitamin A by the body and is a known tumor-fighter.

There are few double-blind studies on chemotherapy.

Very few studies have been carried out to determine if chemotherapy affects survival time in cancer patients beyond a few months.

Although chemotherapy has only proven itself in helping to cure rare cancers like Burkitt's Lymphoma—but is largely ineffective in the big killers: breast, lung, and colon cancers—it is given to almost all cancer patients in order to "orient them toward medical treatment."

Radiation, a known cause of cancer, is given to cancer patients as a form of treatment. This is a case of the medical establishment causing the illness it hopes to cure.

An accepted operation, removal of the ovaries in hysterical women (the ovaries were considered the source of a woman's emotions), was only phased out when psychotherapy became accepted as a treatment for emotional problems at the turn of the century.

Women with a history of breast cancer in their families regularly go into surgery to have their breasts removed as a "prophylactic" measure. This is, to me, the equivalent of having your brain removed because there is a history of mental illness in your family. (Dr. Susan Love rejects this operation, as it is impossible to remove **all** breast tissue.)

Hippocrates, the Father of medicine, forbade surgery in the case of cancer patients because it was harmful.

Surgery is often used when the disease it attempts to treat is not understood.

Some people submit themselves to multiple surgeries in order to assuage their guilt about wanting to hurt others.

Spending hundreds of thousands of dollars on "cutting edge" medical treatments won't necessarily cure you of breast cancer.

Cancer is not a straight-forward progression from tumor to death but can be reversed. This can be done without surgery or drugs.

Inflammatory breast cancer may not be a rare, viscious type of disease, but a stage the body goes through in its self-healing process. The fact that so few women currently live through this disease may be due to "medical interruption," the giving of poisonous chemotherapy drugs to these patients at this crucial time of self-healing.

Doctors can be converted into partners instead of authority figures.

Our attitudes are prime motivators for our body and may determine whether we get sick, stay ill, or get well.

Cancer may begin in infanthood when our mother does not respond to our needs and we learn to hold our irritation within.

Passive cancer patients who "learn to live with the disease" do not survive as long as those with a "fighting spirit."

Cancer can be self-healed in one week by a person with enough spiritual energy who is able to channel it toward getting well.

You can "visualize" away a tumor in your body.

"Spontaneous regression" of cancer, in my opinion, actually involves a lot of hard work. It's the result of the body healing itself.

Breast cancer patients who have a strong network of social support tend to live longer.

Group therapy can enable a terminally-ill breast cancer patient to live on for many years.

A healer can get rid of tumors using only his own bodily energy.

The body, if supported, has almost unlimited healing ability. If the will to live is very strong, most likely a sick person will get well.

You can heal yourself. The mechanisms for healing disease are within your body. Your immune system can be encouraged to work harder.

Getting well can be a profound spiritual experience. It can be a turning point in changing one's life for the better.

The body has a magnificent innate healing ability. Scientists are only now beginning to investigate *cytokines, interleukins,* and *interferons* that are involved with healing wounds and disease. According to Deepak Chopra we manufacture these chemicals in quantity when we feel ecstatic during a pleasurable experience.

Until scientists understand the systems of the body better (they are beginning to find not just one but hundreds of growth factors), trusting and supporting the body to heal itself in a natural way can result in a permanent healing process. The courage to trust the body to heal itself without "medical intervention" or medical interruption is one that can be developed.

Medical intervention in breast cancer is not a proven route to remission or cure.

As for me, I had no desire to surgically remove the symptom of my malaise (i.e., the tumors) as I believed the body created these lumps for a reason. This was the body's way of communicating to me. My body was telling me it could no longer take the stress and negative feelings I was subjecting it to. Merely removing the lump would not touch the underlying causes. I had deep emotional and spiritual problems that were crying out for attention.

The path to wellness is filled with the joy and exhilaration of finding a deep inner-strength. Getting in touch with our innermost being, being honest with ourselves, is a great reward in itself. The gold mine of self-healing is waiting for the self-discoverer. Access is free. All you need is faith, perseverance, and patience. When we have the confidence, when we trust our body and give it the support it needs, the healing systems will activate. Health is only a short time away. We have only to "make the commitment."

Over dinner one evening Kimberly asked, "I wonder what will happen in one hundred years from now? I'd really like to come back to Earth and see if your book has made any difference."

This was the first time she had truly been positive about the work in progress. I was encouraged as I stared off into space imagining a video-tape which began playing before my eyes:

A reporter from the "Los Angeles Times" is interviewing a gynecologist from Glendale, California in the year 2092.

REP: "I've heard there was once an epidemic of a disease called 'breast cancer' and that it was believed that it could be cured with a mutilating amputation of the breast, warfare chemicals, and burning the body with radiation."

GYN: "Yes!" (laughs). "I first read about this strange

obsolete disease and the destructive, expensive method of treatment for it in 'Ripley's Believe It or Not' when I was a boy!"

REP: "Someone told me that the 'treatment' could cost up to three hundred thousand dollars! That was a fortune back then. Do you ever see a case of it these days?"

GYN: "Only very rarely. When we do, we prescribe a course of self-healing that is practically free of cost. First we send the patient to the public library. There she can obtain many excellent manuals about the disease. She can inform herself about detoxification programs, and learn how to de-stress her body in a program that fits her own lifestyle."

REP: "What do these programs consist of, and how do they work?"

GYN: "The newest manuals outline a physical detoxification program consisting of a diet of fresh vegetables and fruits and their freshly prepared juices, soups, whole grains, beans, nuts, and some fish. Vitamins and apricot kernels are also taken. We have the patient slightly undereat for a month to clean out the toxins in an overstressed or poisoned body. We also give patients a free medical pass to the local 'Y' so they can exercise vigorously for at least one hour a day to get a sluggish immune system going. We send them as guests to several group therapy sessions. A spiritual group also teaches them chanting and meditation along with visualization. If they are in a painful, turbulent relationship, we advise them to either change it or break it off. This is of the utmost importance. We like them to be with positive people and develop harmonious relationships."

REP: "What happens then?"

GYN: "If they've done the work, often within a variable period of time, the body will respond with a very intense reaction, a 'flare-up' or 'inflammatory reaction.' The breast turns bright scarlet and heats up in a 'fever' which then kills the cancer cells. This used to be a very terrifying experience until we found it was a process the body goes through to get well. Before detoxification, the body was too weak and toxic, too 'stressed out' to go through this reaction. Because the lymph nodes in the arm are involved, carrying off the cancer cells and disposing of them, the patient has difficulty raising her arm. This reaction does not last long, however. Usually only one or two days. Lymph nodes used to be removed as a routine 'diagnostic' procedure during breast surgery. This left women unprotected in future battles with infections and cancer.

"We've had patients whose tumor completely disappeared within one month after the inflammatory reaction. Of course we advise them to stay on the program for at least seven more months. Even better, for the rest of their lives."

REP: "How did the change in treatment come about?"

GYN: "It happened that one hundred years ago, there was a shift to alternative, holistic medicine. Symptomatic treatment of a part of the body proved fallacious as the whole-person was ill. The mortality rate stayed the same for decades because of a lack of understanding of the disease process. Today the notion of using surgery to cure disease seems rather absurd. We now know that breast cancer involves the decline in health of the **whole body.** We began to look at a person's life, physical, mental, spiritual, and emotional, their relationships with others as well of the general condition of *all* the vital organs in the body instead of focusing on tumors and body parts. Symptomatic treatment was, for the most part, discarded. Some people did respond to surgery, because removing the tumor or the whole breast took some of the toxic load off the liver, which was then able to deal more effectively with all the other toxins in the body. But, in the long run, the majority of women were not helped by it. Often, even after the breast was cut off, the disease metastasized to other parts of the body: the bones, lungs, or brain. Even the eyes. Perhaps it was already there by the time a tumor in the breast became apparent."

REP: "Women who had one or both of their breasts amputated must have looked strange."

GYN: "Well, they had these gel sand-bags or salt-water bags that they would implant inside a woman's skin or even behind a muscle. But the trouble was the silicone sacks leaked or bled, often leading to horrible, painful arthritic problems. Finally, the FDA banned them from the market."

REP: "Isn't it wonderful—women learned to take such

good care of themselves, so that all of them can have healthy, natural breasts for life? Because we have progressed so far in understanding the human body and mind, women can now KEEP THEIR BREASTS!"

Epilogue

Kimberly died February 1, 1993, one week into her thirty-eighth birthday.

Her memorial service was a joyful remembrance. The chapel was packed, testifying to the many lives she had touched. She had been a friend to many and the honest and sincere testimonials that were given contributed to the feeling of intimacy, warmth, and caring with which she blanketed all her friends.

When I rose to speak, I became truly emotional. Kimberly was one of the most beautiful and energetic young women that I ever had the great good fortune to meet. I felt my heart communicating this to the audience and to her spirit which seemed to be ever-present throughout the ceremony.

To say that I will miss her is inadequate. To say that she certainly should not have been at death's door at so young an age is an understatement. I will always remember Kimberly as one of my best friends.

I painted an oil study on paper and a large canvas, "Green Peace," which I dedicated to her. The study was to be auctioned off at Butterfields and Butterfields auction house as a benefit to the Graphic Arts Council for the Los

Angeles County Museum of Art. This was my first participation in a major auction. I invited everyone at the funeral services.

Six years have gone by. Dr. Furr has continued to find **absolutely** no tumors in my body. I have continued to keep up the MOTEP program and work everyday on my immune system. This program has kept me feeling absolutely great. Flu, colds, and allergies are even a thing of the past.

Kimberly fought hard in her own way. She chose the medical route and stuck with it. She is to be commended for her courage. Even in her emaciated condition, she still underwent radiation treatments. The cancer continued to spread into her brain and her intestines. When she did die, it was in a peaceful sleep.

Dedication

I dedicate this book to the memory of my good friend, Kimberly, and to the future of my beautiful niece, Bridget Moss.

Disclaimer

My goal is to present here as much experiential, historical, and scientific information as I can cram into this computer about breast cancer.

It is my hope that the program presented will help all women prevent and/or heal this life-threatening disease.

However, I am not a medical person and, therefore, cannot give medical advice. Any health program or healing therapy should be attempted only under the supervision of a qualified physician and/or gynecologist. The author can assume no responsibility for anyone's health but her own.

Appendix

FORTY-ONE FOODS CONTAINING LAETRILE

(Vitamin B-17)

Used throughout history to kill cancer

cells and prevent cancer.

(Ernest Krebs)

1. Apple seeds
2. Alfalfa sprouts
3. Apricot kernels
   (two-four per day only)
4. Bamboo shoots
5. Barley
6. Beet tops
7. Bitter Almond
8. Blackberries
9. Boysenberries
10. Brewer's Yeast
11. Brown rice
12. Buckwheat
13. Cashews
14. Cherry kernels
15. Cranberries
16. Currants
17. Fava Beans
18. Flax seeds
19. Filberts
20. Garbanzo beans
21. Gooseberries
22. Huckleberries
23. Lentils
24. Lima beans
25. Linseed meal
26. Loganberries
27. Macadamia nuts
28. Millet
29. Millet seed
30. Peach kernels
31. Pecans
32. Plum kernels
33. Quince
34. Raspberries
35. Sorghum Cane Syrup
36. Spinach
37. Sprouts (alfalfa,
    lentil, mung bean,
    buckwheat, garbanzo)
38. Strawberries
39. Walnuts
40. Watercress
41. Yams

Fats and Oils

Crucial to maintaining our health, fats rate a discussion. They are not simply something we must avoid in order to lower our body-fat content, stay or get slim, and lower our risk of heart attacks and cancer.

Omega three fatty acids as well as omega six and nine are needed by the body as well as *some* cholesterol. Our brain, nervous system, hormones, and immune system utilize essential fatty acids and cholesterol as building blocks. Without the essential fatty acids, especially Omega three, we become deficient which may lead to diseases such as cancer.

According to John Finnegan, a nutritional expert on fats and oils, the fats that harm us most are hydrogenated fats such as margarine and solid vegetable shortening that are "plasticized" beyond the point where the body can utilize them as nutrition, and all refined oils. Caged animals also build up more cholesterol than those free to roam, making them less fit for human consumption.

What are "refined oils?" According to Finnegan, in his book *Fats and Oils—A Consumer's Guide* published by Celestial Arts, refined vegetable oils are all oils currently sold in the supermarkets except extra-virgin olive oil! Because of the desire for "shelf life" these oils have been subjected to very high temperatures (up to 500 degrees F.) which creates poisonous trans-fatty acids and damages the vital nutrients in the oils. Refined oils are subjected to processing methods such as deodorization, winterizing, bleaching, and alkali refining that remove most or all of the Vitamin E, lecithin, beta carotene, and essential fatty acids. Trans-fatty acids can contribute to such diseases as blocked arteries leading to heart problems and also cancer. Refined oils are sold in clear glass bottles which allow light to penetrate, causing rancidity. Fresh, expeller pressed oils are fragile and cannot long be exposed to light and air. Most vegetable oils commonly sold for use on salads, for baking, and frying are not only worthless nutritionally and can contribute to consumers becoming deficient in valuable nutrients, they can poison them as well!

In 1987 some small companies in Canada began to produce and bottle expeller-pressed oils without using chemicals or high temperatures, bottling them in dark bottles. Upon opening, the oil should be refrigerated. Finnegan has found the best company that produces oil this way from organic seed: Omega Nutrition which is also distributed by Arrowhead Mills.

In Germany, Dr. Johanna Budwig has used organic flax-seed oil to help her cancer patients get well. Flax-seed oil has the highest content of Omega threes of all oils. It also contains beta carotene and laetrile. Recommended is one to two teaspoons per day.

Eating the right kind of fat can actually help you to lose weight! Omega three and omega six fatty acids stimulate the body's burning of "brown fat" (such as cellulite) and act as a solvent to help the body dissolve and remove hard fats that cause disease.

Obese people are often starving for fats! Eating the right kind of fat will often remove the craving for fatty foods, one of the problems in overeating.

Besides flax seed oil, Omega threes are found in fish. The highest concentrate is found in sardines. Also rich in essential fatty acids are mackerel, salmon, tuna, and trout.

Applying this information to my own program, I now order flax seed oil from Omega Nutrition in Vancouver, Canada. It can be ordered through most health food stores also. I use this oil both on my salads, steamed vegetables, and in spreads for sandwiches in my diet, and have added a massage program using the oil on my body as well as my breasts, alternating it with the fresh lemon. I have found my allergies have disappeared, I never catch whatever flu-bug is going around as I used to always do, and have lump-free breasts with no recurrence of disease. Seeing is believing. Meeting John Finnegan and attending his lectures, I was extremely skeptical. I had thought as the nurse mentioned in the text that "fat is the enemy." The wrong kind of fats, most of the ones readily available to the consumer *are* the enemy. However, good quality, expeller pressed oils can drastically improve health and prevent disease. This has proven the case in my own first-hand experience.

Bibliography

Chapter 2

AIROLA, PAAVA, *Cancer: Causes, Preventions, and Treatment,* Oregon: Sherwood, 1972.

BRINKER, NANCY, *The Race is Run One Step at a Time,* New York: Simon and Schuster, 1990.

BUDOFF, PENNY WISE, M.C., *No More Hot Flashes and Other Good News,* New York: Warner Books, 1984.

COWLES, JANE, *Informed Consent,* New York: Coward, McCann, Georghegan, 1976.

CRILE, GEORGE, JR., M.D., *What Women Should Know About the Breast Cancer Controversy,* New York: Macmillan Publishing Co., 1973.

BOSTON WOMEN'S HEALTH COLLECTIVE, *The New Our Bodies, Ourselves,* New York: Touchstone Book. Simon and Schuster, Inc., 1984.

CURTIS, LINDSAY R., M.D., CURTIS, GLADE, et. al., *My Body—My Decision: What You Should Know About the Most Common Female Surgeries,* Tucson, Arizona: The Body Press, 1986.

EPSTEIN, ALICE HOPPER, *Mind, Fantasy, and Healing—One Woman's Journey from Conflict and Illness to Wholeness and Health,* New York: Delacorte Press, 1989.

HEYDEN, SIEGFRIED, M.D., PITTILLO, ELLEN, Ed.D., *Sensible Talk About Cancer: A Physicians Program for Prevention,* New York: Delair, 1980.

KUSHI, MICHIO and the EAST WEST FOUNDATION, *The Macrobiotic Approach to Cancer,* Wayne, N.J.: Avery Publishing Group, 1981.

KUSHNER, ROSE, *Alternatives: New Developments on the War on Breast Cancer,* Cambridge, Massachusetts: Kensington Press, 1984.

LLOYD, ROBERT, *Dr. Anne's Journal,* Cannon Beach, Oregon: Davar, 1990.

McCAULEY, CAROLE SPEARIN, *Surviving Breast Cancer,* New York: E.P. Dutton, 1979.

SHEEHAN, GEORGE, M.D., *Personal Best,* Emmaus, Pennsylvania: Rodale Press, 1989.

SIMONTON, CARL O., M.D., STEPHANIE MATTHEWS-SIMONTON, CREIGHTON, JAMES, *Getting Well Again,* Toronto: Bantam Books, 1978.

WIGMORE, ANN, *Be Your Own Doctor: Let Living Food Be Your Medicine,* Wayne, New Jersey: Avery, 1982.

Chapter 3

DUKE, MARK, *Acupuncture—The Extraordinary New Book of the Chinese Art of Healing,* New York: Pyramid House, 1972.

GORBACH, SHERWOOD L., M.D., ZIMMERMAN, DAVID R., and WOODS, MARGO, D.S.C., *The Doctor's Anti-Breast-Cancer Diet,* New York: Simon and Schuster, 1984.

LOVE, SUSAN M., M.D., with LINDSEY, KAREN, *Dr. Susan Love's Breast Book,* Reading, Massachusetts: Addison-Wesley, 1990.

MARCHETTI, ALBERT, M.D., *Beating the Odds: Alternative Treatments That Have Worked Miracles Against Cancer,* Chicago: Contemporary Books, 1988.

TERESI, DICK and ADCROFT, PATRICE G., *Omni's Future Medical Almanac,* New York: McGraw-Hill, 1987.

WEBER, MARCEA, *Naturally Sweet Desserts,* Garden City Park, New York: Avery Publishing Group, Inc., 1990.

Chapter 8

GORBACH, SHERWOOD L., M.D., ZIMMERMAN, DAVID R., and WOODS, MARGO, D.S.C., *The Doctor's Anti-Breast-Cancer Diet,* New York: Simon and Schuster, 1984.

LOVE, SUSAN M., M.D., with LINDSEY, KAREN, *Dr. Susan Love's Breast Book,* Reading, Massachusetts: Addison-Wesley, 1990.

MARCHETTI, ALBERT, M.D., *Beating the Odds: Alternative Treatments That Have Worked Miracles Against Cancer,* Chicago: Contemporary Books, 1988.

TERESI, DICK and ADCROFT, PATRICE G., *Omni's Future Medical Almanac,* New York: McGraw-Hill, 1987.

WEBER, MARCEA, *Naturally Sweet Desserts,* Garden City Park, New York: Avery Publishing Group, Inc., 1990.

Chapter 9

GERSON, MAX, M.D., *A Cancer Therapy: Results of Fifty Cases* and *The Cure of Advanced Cancer by Diet Therapy: A Summary of Thirty Years of Clinical Experimentation,* Bonita, CA: Gerson Institute, 1958-1990.

PAULING, LINUS and CAMERON, EWAN, *Cancer and Vitamin C: A Discussion of the Nature, Causes, Prevention, and Treatment of Cancer with Special Reference to the Value of Vitamin C,* Menlo Park, CA: Linus Pauling Institute of Science and Medicine, 1979.

MINDELL, EARL, *Unsafe at Any Meal,* New York, N.Y.: Warner Books, 1987.

SPAIN, JUNE de, *The Little Cyanide Cookbook—Delicious Recipes Rich in Vitamin B17,* Westlake Village, CA: American Media, 1976.

Chapter 10

EVERSON, TILDEN C. and COLE, WARREN, H., *Spontaneous Regression of Cancer,* Philadelphia and London: W.B. Saunders, 1966.

THEMSON, HENRY J., RONAN, ANNE M., et. al., "Effects of Exercise on the Induction of Mammary Carcinogenesis," "Cancer Research" 48: 2720-2723. May 15, 1988.

HOFFMAN, S.A. and HOFFMAN, K.E., PASCHIKIS, et. al., "The Influence of Exercise on the Growth of Transplanted Rat Tumors," "Cancer Patient" 22 (1962) 597-99.

EWING, JAMES, *Causation, Diagnosis, and Treatment of Cancer,* Baltimore, Maryland: Williams and Wilkins Co., 1931. Also from *Beating the Odds,* Marchetti, Albert, M.D., Chicago, Illinois: Contemporary Books, 1988.

Chapter 11

LANDON, MICHAEL, "I Want to See My Kids Grow Up," "Life" magazine, June 1991.

IRELAND, JILL, *Life Wish,* Boston, Toronto: Little Brown, 1987.

"Hell is the Condition of Suffering," "Seiko Times," No. 337: August 1989.

LAWRENCE, CHRIS, M.D., "Reports from Culture Department Representatives," "World Tribune," Monday, Oct. 7, 1991.

GENGERELLI, JOSEPH, KIRKNER, FRANK J., "Psychological Variables in Human Cancer" Symposium. Veterans Hospital, Long Beach, California: October 23, 1953.

PELLETIER, KENNETH R., *Mind as Healer, Mind as Slayer,* New York: Dell, 1977.

Chapter 12

SELYE, HANS, *Stress Without Distress,* Philadelphia and New York: J.B. Lippincott Company, 1974.

LeSHAN, LAWRENCE, Ph.D., *Cancer as a Turning Point,* New York: E.P. Dutton, 1989.

CULLIGAN, MATTHEW J. and SEDLACEK, KEITH, M.D., *How to Avoid Stress Before it Kills You,* New York: Gramercy Publishing Co., 1979.

MARSA, LINDA, "One Last Chance," "Los Angeles Times Magazine," October 20, 1991.

LEVENSON, JAMES and BEMIS, CLAUDIA, M.D., "The Role of Psychological Factors in Cancer Onset and Progression," "Psychosomatics," Vol. 32, #2, Spring 1991.

SKLAR, "Science," Vol. 205, No. 4405, August 1979.

LEVY, S. and HERBERMAN, R., et. al., "Journal of Clinical Oncology," Vol. 5, #3, Mar. 1978.

IDEKA, DIASOLKU, "Seikyo Times," Dec. 1987: p. 32.

PELETIER, KENNETH, *Mind as Healer, Mind as Slayer,* New York: Dell, 1977.

Chapter 13

COUSINS, NORMAN, *Head First, the Biology of Hope,* New York: E.P. Dutton, 1989. pp. 118-119.

CUTLER, MAX, "Psychological Variables in Human Cancer" Symposium. Veterans Hospital, Long Beach, CA: Oct. 23, 1953.

GRAHAM, BARBARA, "Mind/Body Medicine," "Vogue," Sept. 1991.

LANDON, MICHAEL, "I Want to See My Kids Grow Up," "Life" magazine. June 1991. pp. 24-32.

LEVENSON, FREDERICK B., DR., *The Causes and Prevention of Cancer,* New York: Stein and Day, 1985.

JAMISON, ROBERT N., BURISH, THOMAS G., and WALLSTON, KENNETH A., "Psychogenic Factors in Predicting Survival of Breast Cancer Patients," "Journal of Clinical Oncology," May 1987: pp. 768-782.

MENNINGER, KARL, *Man Against Himself,* New York: Harcourt, Brace, 1938.

IRELAND, JILL, *Life Wish,* Boston: Little Brown, 1987.

JENSEN, MORGANS R., "Psychobiological Factors Predicting the Course of Breast Cancer," "Journal of Personality," June 1955: pp. 317-42.

WEISMAN, A.D., WORDEN, J.W., "Psychosocial Analysis of Cancer Deaths," "Omega," 6 1975: pp. 61-75.

Index

— N —

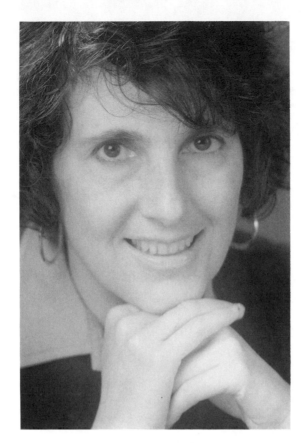

About the Author

Susan Moss began saving lives as a teenager working as a lifeguard.

At the University of Nevada she graduated with honors receiving a B.A. in Art and Psychology. She helped establish a Suicide Prevention Clinic in 1966, with Dr. James B. Nichols, which is still in operation today.

After further study at Otis Art Institute, she became an exhibiting artist worldwide, included in both public and private collections such as: Los Angeles County Museum, ARCO, IBM, Robert A. Rowan, and James Coburn.

Her work can be seen at Forum Gallery, New York City, New York; Ruth Bachofner Gallery, Santa Monica, California; Bobbie Greenfield, Venice, California; Manny Silverman Gallery, Los Angeles, California.

Some of the characters in her gene pool include Art Dealers Frank and Klaus Perls, Psychologist Fritz Perls, Artist Max Ernst, as well as many women physicians.

KEEP YOUR
BREASTS!

PREVENTING BREAST CANCER THE NATURAL WAY

by Susan Moss

KEEP YOUR
BREASTS!

PREVENTING BREAST CANCER THE NATURAL WAY

by Susan Moss

$19.95 u.s. 25.00 can
Add $ 3.00 for shipping & handling
(california residents add sales tax)

name

address

ENCLOSE CHECK OR MONEY ORD
TO Susan Moss
4767 York Boulevard
Los Angeles, California 90042
213.255.3382

phone

KEEP YOUR
BREASTS!

PREVENTING BREAST CANCER THE NATURAL WAY

by Susan Moss

$19.95 u.s. 25.00 can
Add $ 3.00 for shipping & handling
(california residents add sales tax)

name

address

ENCLOSE CHECK OR MONEY ORDE
TO Susan Moss
4767 York Boulevard
Los Angeles, California 90042
213.255.3382

phone